Easy
KETO
Cooking

EMBRACE THE KETO LIFESTYLE
WITH OVER 100 SATISFYING
AND DELICIOUS RECIPES

13-Digit ISBN: 978-1-60433-883-6
10-Digit ISBN: 1-60433-883-0

This book may be ordered by mail from the publisher. Please include $5.99 for postage and handling. Please support your local bookseller first!

Books published by Cider Mill Press Book Publishers are available at special discounts for bulk purchases in the United States by corporations, institutions, and other organizations. For more information, please contact the publisher.

Cider Mill Press Book Publishers
"Where good books are ready for press"
PO Box 454
12 Spring Street
Kennebunkport, Maine 04046
Visit us online!
cidermillpress.com

Typography: Bushcraft, Fenwick Park JF, Helvetica Rounded, Neutraface 2 Text, Sentinel, Hello Beautiful
See page 269 for list of recipes and photographs courtesy of Sahil Makhija.

Printed in China
1 2 3 4 5 6 7 8 9 0
First Edition

Easy
KETO
Cooking

**EMBRACE THE KETO LIFESTYLE
WITH OVER 100 SATISFYING
AND DELICIOUS RECIPES**

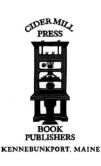

CIDER MILL PRESS

BOOK
PUBLISHERS
KENNEBUNKPORT, MAINE

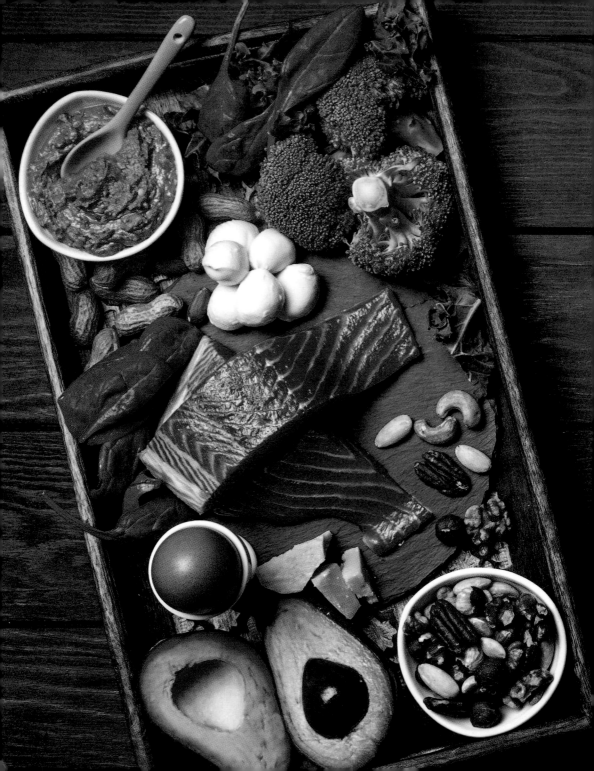

Contents

Introduction

Welcome to the ketogenic diet—keto, for short—which is a high-fat, adequate-protein, low-carb way of eating. It turns your body into a fat-burning machine, fine-tuning your metabolism to burn your body's years of stored-up fat. What this does is reset your understanding of food, and help you use what you eat to improve your energy levels and mood, regulate hormones, stabilize your blood sugar levels, enhance your mental clarity, and lose weight, of course. But weight loss is only one of its many incidental benefits.

UNLEARN EVERYTHING

For decades now, we've been told that fat is bad, that saturated fats are responsible for raising cholesterol and bringing on heart disease, which had become a sort of epidemic in America by the 1970s. The "diet-heart hypothesis," introduced in the 1980s, linked fat to bad health based on a few animal studies (none of which were carried out on humans) and passed into public policy even before research was complete and before the studies had drawn any solid conclusions. The result? Fat became the enemy. Butter was replaced by margarine. Red meat was off the table and replaced by poultry, without skin, because that's where all the "bad" saturated fats hid. Full-fat milk and milk products gave way to watery skim milk. Granola became a buzzword. A new health fad had begun—low-fat everything.

Yet heart disease continues unabated; as of this year, one in three deaths in the U.S. is attributed to cardiovascular disease. Diabetes has skyrocketed, from 2.39 million people diagnosed in 1965 to 23.35 million people in 2015, with about 7 million more undiagnosed cases. Something was clearly wrong with the low-fat approach.

In the meantime, nutrition research caught up. More and more medical studies have disproved the role of fat and cholesterol in heart disease. Long-term reviews found little difference in longevity between people over 60 with high and low LDL cholesterol. Instead, focus shifted to the role of processed carbs and sugar in our diet, both of which are found in abundance in the so-called "health food" being peddled by brands everywhere. It turns out we were looking at the wrong bad guy all this time.

So fat is our friend. Why? Fat is more energy-dense than carbohydrates—gram for gram, fat has more calories than carbs (9 calories per gram as opposed to 4 calories per gram of carbs). Carbs are broken down faster, finding their way into your system quicker, while fats burn slower and more evenly over a longer period of time, giving you a stabler source of energy. When you eat refined carbs and sugars, the super-quick breakdown spikes your insulin, causing a sharp rise—and subsequent crash—in your energy levels. This yo-yoing of energy leaves you feeling drained and fatigued. Cut out carbs, and your body turns to its own fat for energy, which is the whole point of the keto diet. But it can take significant deprogramming to learn to love fats after being conditioned to believe that they're bad for you. How do you get there faster? By cooking and eating tasty, healthy, high-fat food that will make you feel at your optimum. That is the essence of what this book is all about.

LIFESTYLE, NOT DIET

The key to embracing the keto way of eating is to think of it as a lifestyle and not a diet. While you are cutting out grains, sugars, and processed carbs, you're not cutting out food. Instead, you're encouraged to eat your fill and to eat well. How could you possibly feel like you're on a restricted diet when you're tucking into a Mushroom and Swiss Cheese Frittata (page 41), Grilled Garlic Calamari (page 65), Bouillabaisse (page 134), or Grilled Lemon Haddock with Basil-Walnut Pesto (page 220)? The recipes in this book span the spectrum from familiar comfort foods and family favorites to party nibbles. What's more, each recipe comes with exact serving sizes and macros, so you can take the guesswork out of the equation and focus on the important bit—enjoying the food.

And that's the other great thing about the ketogenic diet: so long as you're getting your fix of fats and proteins, you'll never be hungry. Hunger is the biggest hurdle in any diet, and most diets that focus on restricting calories or food intake leave you feeling dissatisfied and, consequently, "hangry." Hunger can also make you go off your diet a lot faster. Not on keto. Proteins and fats are the components of food that keep you sated longer, so not only are you not reaching for diet-breaking snacks, but you're also not turning into a hangry monster between meals.

So, then, is keto all about eating bacon and butter at every meal? Not at all. Keto is all about eating real food: good fats, healthy proteins, and carbs derived from fresh greens and veggies. Don't fear the carbs in vegetables; most above-ground vegetables have fairly low glycemic indices that won't trigger an insulin spike. You want to avoid root vegetables and tubers like beetroot and potatoes—by nature they're full of the starches that the plant needs to grow, which are not keto-conducive. A lot of keto dieters will tell you that you can't eat more than 20 grams of carbs a day; this is not always true. Everyone has a different carb tolerance and while some people can eat up to 50 grams of carbs and stay in ketosis, some will get kicked out if they go over 30 grams. The trick is to find your sweet spot.

The truth, though, is that keto doesn't require overthinking. It's easy and, trust us, it's the most enjoyable way of dieting you'll ever try. When you're feeling as good as you do on keto, it stops becoming that dreaded word—diet—and instead becomes a lifestyle you'll want to sustain for, well, life. So ditch those carbs, make friends with fat, and enjoy the journey to great health on keto.

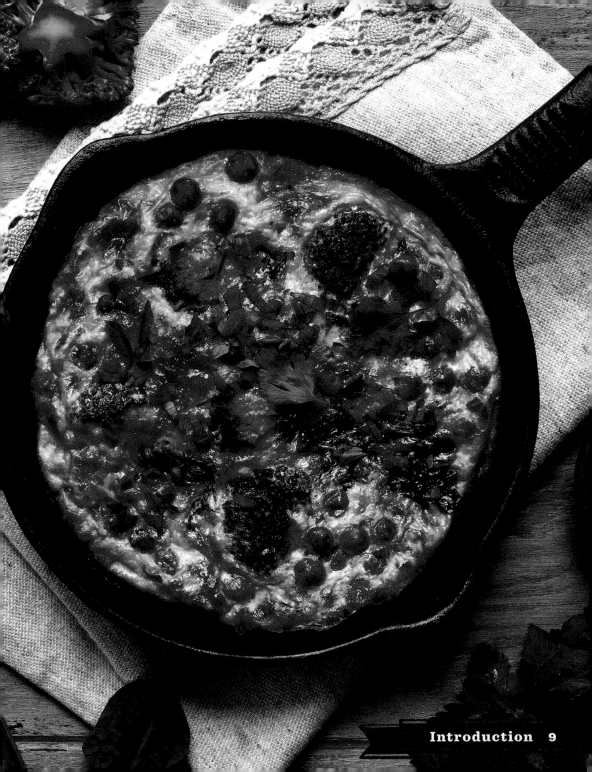

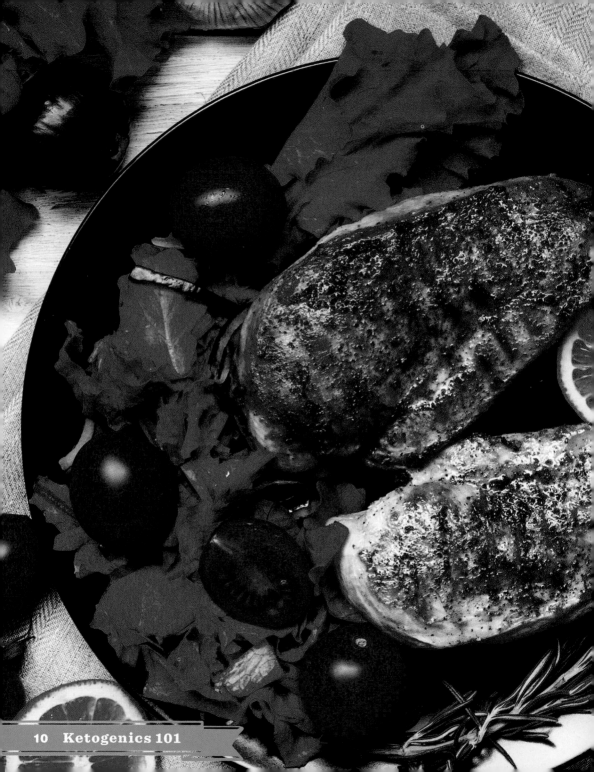

Ketogenics 101

WHAT IS KETOSIS?

The ketogenic diet goes by many names—low-carb high fat (LCHF), low-carb, keto—but at the heart of it the concept remains the same: deprive your body of carbs so it can turn to fat and stored body fat for energy through a process called "ketosis."

Normally, our bodies use glucose as their primary source of energy, derived through the carbohydrates we eat. On the keto diet, we deprive our body of these carbs by limiting our consumption of them to under 20 to 30 grams in a day, or to roughly 5% of our total intake of food. When this happens, our body has to find an alternate source of fuel to keep us going, and that is where ketosis kicks in and our body starts to use fat for energy. The liver converts fatty acids into ketone bodies that the brain and other organs can use as fuel.

WHAT'S SO GREAT ABOUT KETO?

Well, for starters, keto effectively turns your body into a fat-burning machine, making it a great way to lose weight, while also lowering your overall body fat. But you don't need to have a weight problem to be following the keto diet—a lot of people find that it gives them greater mental clarity, lowers cholesterol and blood pressure, and keeps them away from processed and sugar-heavy foods that have now been shown to be the cause many diseases.

When you eat high fat and moderate protein, you will also find that you are satiated and satisfied with your meals. Not craving those between-meal snacks is half the battle!

The keto diet has also been known to be very effective in helping people who suffer from diabetes, epilepsy, and a number of other autoimmune diseases. In fact, keto is not new—it was actually formulated for epilepsy patients and was found to greatly reduce the frequency and intensity of seizures. We're only now realizing the many other benefits that come from following the keto lifestyle.

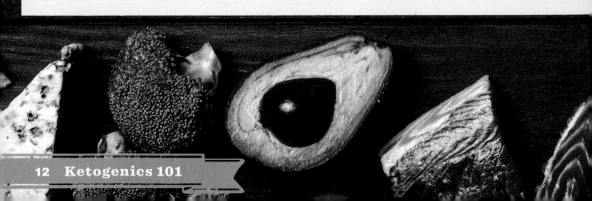

WHAT, EXACTLY, IS THE ROLE OF INSULIN IN KETO?

If you've been eating carbs, you're probably familiar with the post-lunch slump, that hour or two when your energy dips after you eat rice, bread, or pasta for lunch. That is due to the insulin in your body regulating the metabolism of carbohydrates and fats. After a carb-heavy meal, your pancreas produces insulin to help break down the glucose and convert it into glycogen that your body can use for energy. The insulin also triggers the production of serotonin and melatonin, which calms you down and induces sleep.

But insulin is also the hormone that converts excess glycogen to body fat when your body has more carbs than it needs. When you eat carb- and sugar-heavy foods meal after meal, your insulin levels remain high for extended periods of time. Eventually, over time, your cells are unable to use the insulin effectively, leading to insulin resistance, which has been implicated in the rise of type 2 diabetes and many other autoimmune diseases.

On keto, with your carb levels so low, your glucose levels aren't elevated, and your insulin doesn't spike after a meal. Lower insulin levels mean greater insulin sensitivity, cutting down on metabolic disorders and leading to effective fat burning. As a plus, you'll find you have greater mental clarity and a more stable level of energy throughout the day.

WHAT ARE MACROS AND WHY DO THEY MATTER?

"Macros" is short for "macronutrients," which is the breakdown of the components of your food. These include carbohydrates, proteins, and fats—the three components that you should keep track of on keto. Macros can be tracked through fitness apps like MyFitnessPal or Lose It.

On a keto diet, it's important to monitor your daily macros, to ensure you're getting enough fat and just enough carbs. Ideally you could look at 70 to 75%

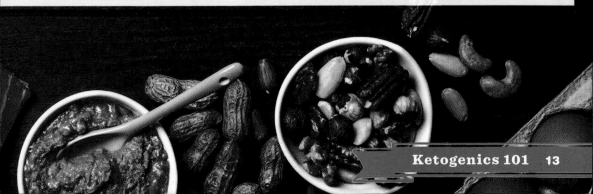

of your daily calories coming from fat sources, 20 to 25% from protein, and 5 to 10% from carbohydrates, specifically net carbs. This is what will keep your body in ketosis and fat-burning mode.

WHAT ARE NET CARBS?

Most foods containing carbs have a dietary fiber or roughage component. Fiber is important for the body, because it helps with the absorption of nutrients in your gut and regulates bowel movements. A lot of dietary fiber is also insoluble and passes through your gut without being digested, so it doesn't count towards your total carb intake. Simply put, net carbs are the total amount of carbs in your food, minus the fiber. On keto, you want to keep your net carb intake between 5 to 10%.

WHAT KIND OF CARBOHYDRATES SHOULD MY 5 TO 10% COMPRISE OF?

When it comes to consuming carbs on the keto diet, you want those to come largely from vegetables, specifically green, leafy vegetables like spinach, kale, lettuce, chard, etc. Cruciferous vegetables like cauliflower and broccoli are high in fiber, and zucchini and eggplant are also sources of good carbs. You want to avoid starchy veggies like potatoes, sweet potatoes, and corn—these are likely to kick you out of ketosis with just a mouthful. More colorful veggies like peppers, tomatoes, and red onions can be consumed, but they're best eaten in moderation. It's also possible that some of your carbs might come from dairy products like cheese, so you want to read those labels carefully. All grains and grain products are off the table. You want to be especially careful with store-bought sauces and even mayonnaise—it's amazing how many hidden carbs they can have.

SO, WHAT SHOULD I BE EATING ON KETO?

Apart from the vegetables mentioned earlier, there is a whole lot to eat on the keto diet. When it comes to protein sources, you can pretty much eat any kind of meat. This includes poultry like chicken, duck, turkey, and quail; red meats like beef, lamb, pork, and venison; and also eggs of all kinds. High-fat dairy products like cream, cheese, butter, and full-fat yogurt (in moderation) are all keto friendly, though you want to avoid milk itself as its carb count is high. Nuts are a great source of good fats, especially macadamia nuts, hazelnuts, almonds, and walnuts, but you want to be careful about eating peanuts and carb-heavy cashews in large quantities. That is why tracking macros so you can keep tabs on your overall carb intake is so important.

Now, since sugar is completely off the table on keto, it eliminates most fruits from the diet. However, there are a few that fall into the keto-friendly category—mainly avocadoes, and berries such as strawberries, raspberries, and blackberries. Once again, it's important to consume these in moderation in keeping with your macros.

Fats, the largest component of your diet, can come from both plant and animal sources. When choosing meat, choose fattier cuts, and eat poultry with the skin on, since that's where a lot of the fat is. The other sources of pure fat are your oils, healthy ones like olive, coconut, and avocado, besides ghee and butter. Animal fats like lard, bacon grease, and duck fat are not only healthy, but also add some serious flavor to your food.

HOW DO I KNOW WHEN I'M IN KETOSIS?

Ketosis is the state your body is in when it switches from a carb-burning to a fat-burning mechanism. In this state, your liver is actively converting fats into ketones, and these can be tracked using ketone detection strips. These strips measure the number of ketones you excrete, though that's not always an accurate measure. There are also blood ketone monitors and breath monitors, both of which are expensive and, frankly, unnecessary. The most important thing to do is to listen to your body and focus on the food and the nutrition you're getting.

There are also some symptoms—called the keto flu—that mark the transition into ketosis as your body adapts to the new diet, but not everyone experiences it the same way.

WHAT IS THE KETO FLU?

As your body makes its transition from burning carbs to burning fat, it takes a few days to adapt. This can vary anywhere between 3 to 15 days depending on your body, metabolism, and insulin sensitivity. In these early days, it's not uncommon to feel a sense of malaise, some fatigue, and occasionally headaches. This is also due to the loss of electrolytes since the keto diet can be diuretic. Carbs hold on to water, and as you reduce your carb intake, your body's water retention also reduces. But don't let the keto flu scare you; it fades within a couple of days. The best way to combat it is by consuming electrolyte-rich items like soup or chicken stock; even a bouillon cube in water will work in a pinch. Most people, though, won't experience the flu at all, and will be able to transition into ketosis effortlessly.

CAN I HAVE A CHEAT DAY ON KETO?

Unlike other diets, keto is an all or nothing process. Eat too many carbs and you'll kick yourself right out of ketosis, and you'll have to begin the process of getting into it all over again. As a rule, it's best not to cheat at all, at least in the first month of the diet.

But as your body becomes adapted, you'll find it's easier to slip into ketosis, at which point the occasional cheat day won't hurt. They've actually been known to break a weight-loss stall after a few months of keto adaptation.

And though the idea of a cheat day may sound great, you'll often find that going back to processed carbs and sugar actually makes you more miserable than happy. You want to cheat responsibly, and not turn a cheat meal into a cheat day, and a cheat day into a cheat week. Cheat rarely, and cheat well, perhaps throwing complex carbs and whole grain food into your day, instead of diving headfirst into a bag of chips or a tub of ice cream.

IS ALCOHOL ALLOWED ON THE KETO DIET?

Ideally, alcohol is best avoided, as it can hamper weight loss irrespective of the diet you are on. However, occasionally you may find yourself in a social situation where you can't (or don't want to) turn down a drink. Are there keto-safe drinks? Yes. Most distilled spirits, like whiskey, white rum, cognac, vodka, and tequila are virtually carb-free. You want to be careful with dark rum, because it can contain a significant amount of sugar. Sweet liqueurs and beers are total no-nos (even the light beers have enough carbs to swallow up your entire day's allowance), as are sugared sodas. If you must cut your drink, pick sugar-free sodas and mixers. And while you can indulge in a glass or two of dry red or white wine, it's best not to exceed that amount, given that, on average, a glass of wine contains close to 3 grams of carbs.

It's also important to note that on keto, as the alcohol is likely to hit you much quicker and harder and hangovers can be significantly worse because you don't have carbs to buffer it with, it's essential to drink plenty of water with your alcohol. The most important thing to remember, though, is that alcohol adds empty calories to your diet, so weigh your choices carefully.

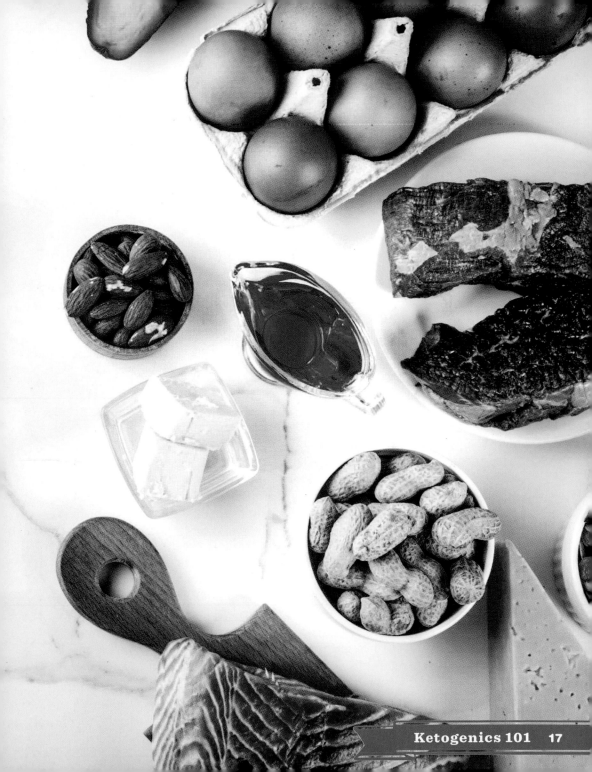

The Keto Dos and Don'ts

DON'T THINK OF KETO AS A MAGIC DIET

While the keto diet does turn your body into a fat-burning machine, it's important to not think it will magic away fat overnight. Yes, the keto diet works faster and more visibly than some other diets, and you may lose more initial weight with it, but it's important to exercise control and stick to your macros to see results. The initial, very quick weight drop is often just water weight, so it's normal to find your weight stalling and weight loss slowing a bit after the first few pounds. It's also important to realize that everybody is unique, so the diet will work differently for different people.

DON'T OBSESS OVER THE SCALE

Often, people get too caught up with the weighing scale. Keto is so much more than a number on a scale; it impacts how you feel and your overall well-being. Sometimes people lose inches rather than weight while on keto; often, your body is losing fat and gaining muscle. There are various reasons the numbers

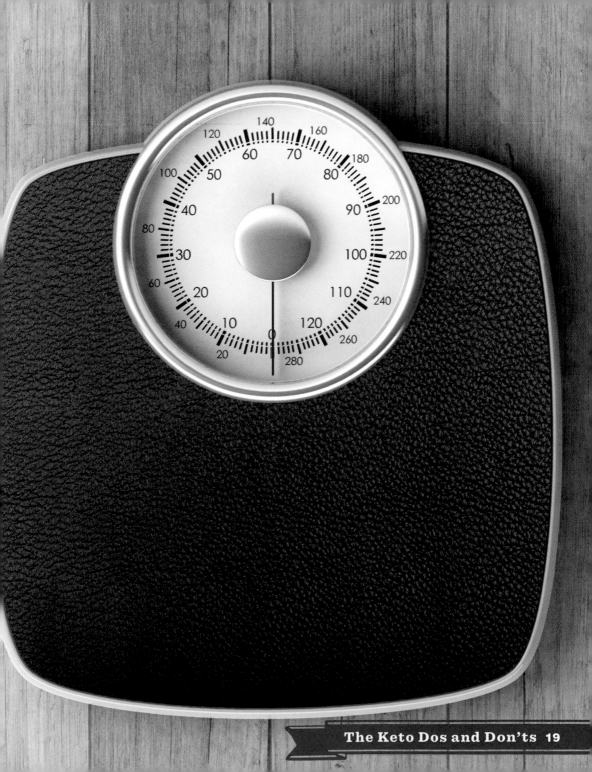

on the scale may not drop, but if you are feeling good, losing inches, and overall getting the benefits of being on keto, it's best to keep the scale obsession to a minimum.

DO EAT LOTS OF REAL FOOD

On the keto diet (and in life in general) it's important to eat good quality food. Fresh vegetables, meat, and dairy are so much healthier than their packaged and processed counterparts. If you eat good food, you will feel good.

DO COUNT YOUR MACROS

Being committed and having discipline definitely yields better results. It's very important to know how much you are eating and whether you are getting the right amount of fats, protein, and carbs from the food you eat. If you aren't hitting your macros, there's a chance you'll be left hungry and craving unhealthy food. Plus, monitoring your macros makes for steadier weight loss. We've included the nutritional info by serving to make it easier for you to keep track of your macros on a meal-by-meal basis.

DRINK LOTS OF WATER

This cannot be stressed enough. It's extremely important to stay hydrated and drink plenty of water while you are on the keto diet. Since your body is not holding on to any water, you need to keep your reserves replenished. Drink at least $1/2$ gallon a day, if not more. And if you don't fancy plain water, it's amazing what a slice of lime or a few cucumber slices can do to the taste.

DON'T OVEREAT

While there is a lot of debate about whether calories matter on this diet, it's important to realize that if you stuff your face and overeat, no matter what diet you're on, it won't work. If you are eating more food than your body requires, you're not helping it shed weight.

DON'T EAT PROCESSED OR PACKAGED FOOD

Most processed food isn't good for you. There's significant deterioration in the quality of macronutrients when food is overprocessed and packaged food always has a lot of insidious, hidden carbs. It's best to eat as much fresh produce as possible and cook most, if not all, of your own food. Also, processed or packaged foods like peanut butter and mayonnaise, which are keto friendly, are still best made on your own, as most supermarket brands will include sugar or ingredients like palm oil that you want to avoid.

DO CHECK THE NUTRITIONAL INFO OF ALL FOOD YOU EAT

Always check the nutritional labels on items before you eat them; it's important to check the nutritional label for carb content as well as for the full list of ingredients. Even with fresh produce like vegetables, if you find yourself in doubt, a quick search on the internet can help you find the nutritional information for the item. It's always better to be safe than sorry.

DO USE NATURAL, SUGAR-FREE OPTIONS

When it comes to sugar-free sweeteners, it can get pretty confusing because there are currently a lot of different options in the market. Some of these are keto safe, like erythritol and stevia. Most others are best avoided, as they either have a high glycemic index, which can cause

your insulin to spike, or are just generally deemed unhealthy. Sugar alcohols like maltitol and xylitol have high glycemic indexes and are not advised. Natural sugars like coconut sugar, agave nectar, and even honey trigger insulin just like white sugar, so they're completely off the table on this diet. It's not a big deal if you drink a diet soda with aspartame once in a while, but it's best to try and stick to more natural sugar substitutes like stevia.

DON'T GO OVERBOARD ON THE FAT

For some reason, when people think high-fat, they assume it's eating sticks of butter. This couldn't be further from the truth. Not only is it important to incorporate good fat sources into your diet, but when it comes to weight loss, it's also important to have an overall calorie deficit so your body can burn its own fat for fuel.

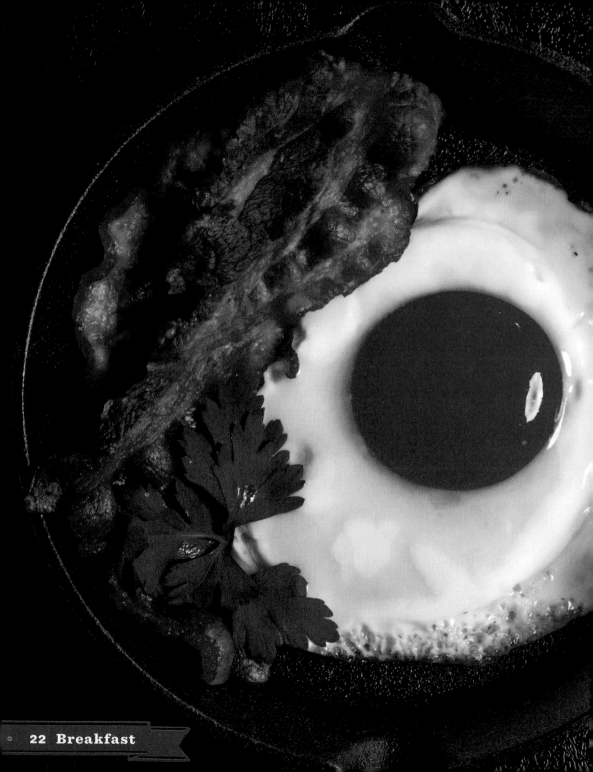

Breakfast

Nothing gets you up and out of bed like the thought of a good breakfast. On keto, you can really indulge yourself for breakfast—think eggs, ham, cheese, and bacon. Eggs, you will discover, are your keto best friends, packed full of good fats and highly nutritious—and it helps that they're so versatile. Other than all the poaching, scrambling, and frying they lend themselves to, they're also great vehicles for leftovers—you can make a frittata out of random ingredients in your refrigerator, be it leftover roast chicken, sautéed vegetables, or even meatloaf scraps. Eggs are a blank canvas for you to paint your culinary skills upon.

On the ketogenic diet, breakfast goes a long way toward getting a good portion of your fats and proteins in. Not only does it add significantly to your daily macros, it also keeps you satiated, so hunger pangs don't kick in and have you reaching for that rogue mid-morning cookie. These recipes are easily customizable, so feel free to add in whatever you fancy (whatever fits in the ketogenic diet, that is). Just be sure not to skip breakfast; it's the fastest way to a happy keto day.

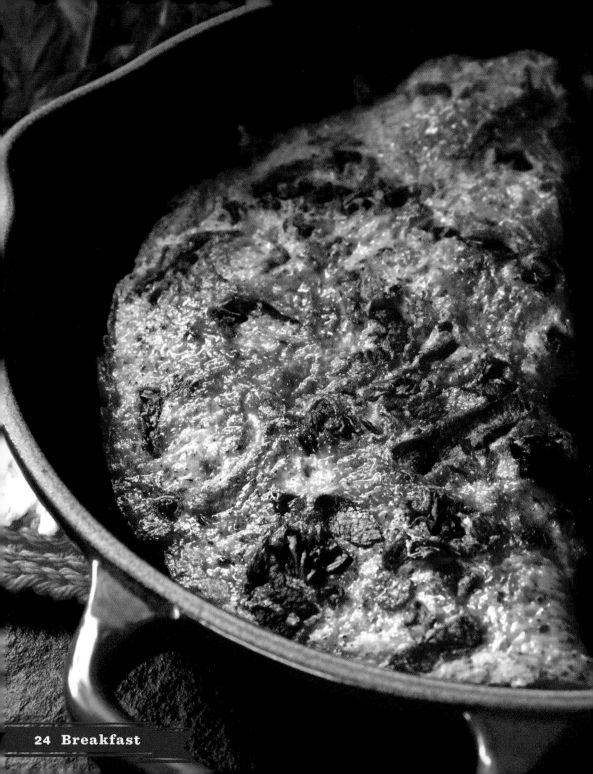

Bacon and Cheese Omelet

YIELD: 1 SERVING • PREP TIME: 5 MINUTES • COOK TIME: 10 MINUTES
NUTRITIONAL INFO: CALORIES: 368 • FAT: 32G • NET CARBS: 1G • PROTEIN: 17G

Bacon and an egg always make for a good breakfast.

1 Add the bacon to a cold pan. Turn the burner to medium and allow the bacon fat to render out. Add the basil to the hot pan and fry along with the bacon.

2 Beat the egg, season with salt and pepper, and add to the hot pan.

3 Sprinkle on the cheese and fold the omelet. Once cooked, remove and serve.

INGREDIENTS

2 strips bacon, chopped

1 tablespoon basil leaves, chopped

1 egg

Salt and pepper, to taste

1 tablespoon cheddar cheese

Baked Eggs with Zucchini, Green Pepper, and Plum Tomato

YIELD: 4 SERVINGS • PREP TIME: 10 MINUTES • COOK TIME: 1½ TO 2 HOURS
NUTRITIONAL INFO: CALORIES: 326 • FAT: 28G • NET CARBS: 5G • PROTEIN: 14G

Save this for the summer, when you can step away and enjoy the morning with a cup of coffee.

INGREDIENTS

- 2 tablespoons olive oil
- ½ onion, chopped fine
- 1 small zucchini, chopped
- 1 small green pepper, seeded and chopped
- 1 plum tomato, chopped
- ¼ cup chopped fresh basil
- 8 eggs
- ½ cup heavy cream
- Salt and pepper, to taste

1 Lightly grease the inside of the slow cooker with a teaspoon of oil. In large skillet, warm the remaining oil and then cook the onion, zucchini, and green pepper until just tender, about 5 minutes. Add the tomato and basil and stir to heat through. Remove from heat.

2 In a large bowl, beat the eggs and heavy cream until well mixed. Add the vegetable mixture and stir until combined. Pour the eggs and vegetables into the slow cooker, season with salt and pepper, cover, and turn on Low. Cook for 1 to 2 hours, until eggs are thoroughly cooked. To test for doneness, insert a clean knife in the center. If it comes out clean, the dish is ready.

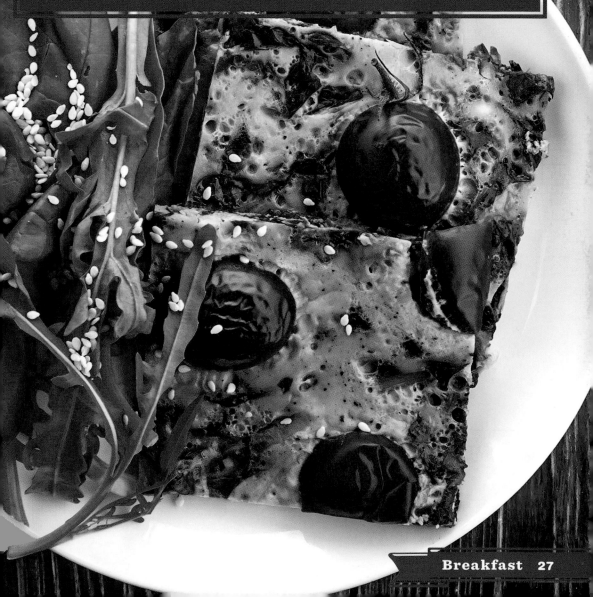

NOTE: CREATE A GOURMET LOW-CARB VERSION OF EGGS BENEDICT BY SERVING THIS YUMMY EGG DISH ON TOP OF A SLICE OF TOASTED KETO BREAD WITH A PIECE OF GRILLED CANADIAN BACON AND A DOLLOP OF HOMEMADE HOLLANDAISE SAUCE. WHEN THE BAKED EGGS HAVE ABOUT A HALF HOUR LEFT, MAKE THE HOLLANDAISE SAUCE BY WHISKING 3 EGG YOLKS WITH 1 TABLESPOON EACH WATER AND LEMON JUICE IN A SMALL SAUCEPAN UNTIL WELL COMBINED. PUT THE SAUCEPAN OVER LOW HEAT AND KEEP MIXING, COOKING FOR ABOUT 5 MINUTES UNTIL MIXTURE GETS FROTHY AND LIGHT. REMOVE THE PAN FROM THE HEAT AND STIR IN 6 TABLESPOONS OF BUTTER, ONE AT A TIME. SEASON WITH SALT AND PEPPER AND A DASH OF CAYENNE.

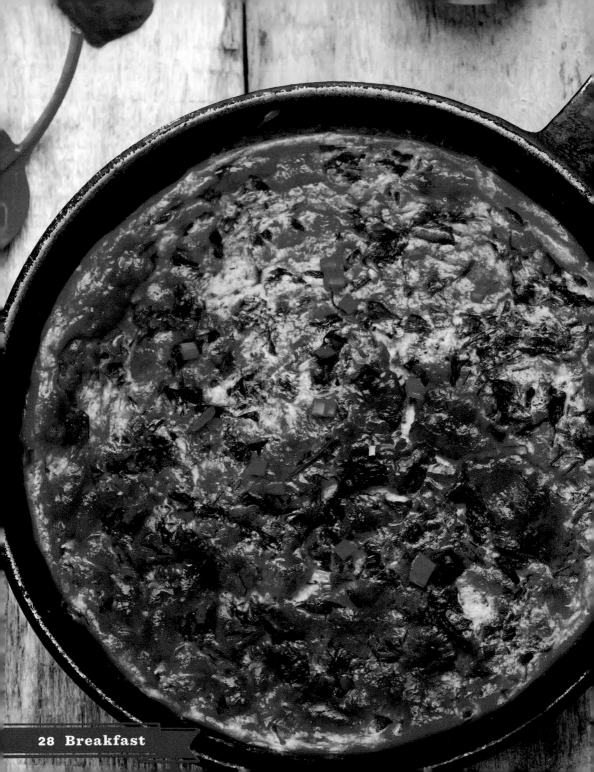

Eggs with Ham and Spinach

YIELD: 2 SERVINGS • PREP TIME: ABOUT 5 MINUTES • COOK TIME: 1 HOUR
NUTRITIONAL INFO: CALORIES: 573 • FAT: 48G • NET CARBS: 6G • PROTEIN: 30G

This triple-threat breakfast is the perfect choice for hitting your morning macros out of the park, not to mention the incredible flavor.

1 In a small skillet, heat the oil over medium-high heat. Add the ham, coat with oil, and brown slightly, about a minute. Remove from heat.

2 In a large bowl, beat the eggs with the heavy cream until well blended. Add the spinach and parsley and whisk to combine everything well, being sure to break up the spinach pieces.

3 Place the ham in the slow cooker and pour the egg mixture over the top. Cover and cook on Low for about 1 hour, until the eggs are cooked through. Season with salt and pepper and serve.

INGREDIENTS

1 tablespoon olive oil

3½ oz. cooked ham, cut into pieces

6 eggs

½ cup heavy cream

½ cup steamed spinach, chopped, excess water squeezed out

2 tablespoons fresh parsley, chopped

Salt and pepper, to taste

Bell Pepper and Broccoli Frittata

YIELD: 4 SERVINGS • PREP TIME: 5 MINUTES
COOK TIME: 1 HOUR TO 2 HOURS 15 MINUTES
NUTRITIONAL INFO: CALORIES: 282 • FAT: 22G • NET CARBS: 4G • PROTEIN: 15G

Broccoli is loaded with Vitamin C and dietary fiber.

INGREDIENTS

2 tablespoons extra virgin olive oil

4 tablespoons onion, chopped

2 garlic cloves, minced

½ red or green bell pepper, seeds and ribs removed, thinly sliced

8 large eggs

4 tablespoons heavy cream

2 tablespoons fresh chopped parsley

1 tablespoon fresh thyme

¾ cup fresh broccoli florets, cut into bite-sized pieces

1 Heat the oil in a skillet and add the onion, garlic, and bell pepper. Cook over medium-high heat until onion is translucent, about 3 minutes.

2 In a large bowl, whisk eggs with heavy cream, then add herbs and broccoli pieces. Add the cooked vegetables. Take a large piece of parchment paper, fold it in half, and place it in the slow cooker so it comes up the sides of the cooker. This will give you a way to lift out the egg dish once it is cooked. Pour the egg mixture on top of the parchment paper.

3 Cover and cook on High for about 1 hour or on Low for close to 2 hours until eggs are set.

4 Run a spatula along the sides of the cooker to loosen the parchment paper. Use the paper to lift the frittata out of the cooker and slide it onto a serving plate.

Scrambled Eggs with Cheese

YIELD: 2 SERVINGS • PREP TIME: 5 MINUTES • COOK TIME: 5 MINUTES
NUTRITIONAL INFO: CALORIES: 728 • FAT: 63G • NET CARBS: 3G • PROTEIN: 38G

This is gooey goodness at its best. Well, you could always add bacon crumbles to take it way over the top, but the egg-and-cheese combo is pretty darn perfect in its simplicity.

1 Heat a skillet over medium-high heat. Melt the butter in the skillet, being careful not to let it burn.

2 In a bowl, whisk the eggs until combined. Add the cream and whisk it into the eggs. Pour the egg mixture into the hot skillet. Using a wooden spoon, stir the eggs in the skillet as they start to cook. After a couple of minutes, turn the heat down to medium. Top the eggs with the cheese and stir it in as the eggs finish cooking. Be careful not to overcook the eggs.

3 Remove from heat, add salt and pepper, and serve immediately.

INGREDIENTS

2 tablespoons butter

6 large eggs

¼ cup heavy cream

1 cup shredded sharp cheddar cheese

Salt and pepper, to taste

Spinach and Mushroom Egg Bake

YIELD: 6 SERVINGS • PREP TIME: 15 MINUTES • COOK TIME: 1 TO 2½ HOURS
NUTRITIONAL INFO: CALORIES: 371 • FAT: 30G • NET CARBS: 5G • PROTEIN: 18G

This is delicious alongside fresh salsa. Chop 2 very ripe tomatoes and put them in a small bowl. Add a squirt of lime juice, a tablespoon of finely minced onion, 1 clove of crushed garlic, and a teaspoon or so of chopped jalapeño pepper (or a spicy pepper of your choice) to a bowl and mix. Season with pepper and just a dash of salt and serve.

INGREDIENTS

2 tablespoons extra virgin olive oil

1 cup onion,
chopped fine

1 cup sliced mushrooms of choice

4 cups spinach leaves, coarse
stems removed, leaves ripped or
cut into smaller pieces

12 eggs

1 cup heavy cream

1 tablespoon chopped fresh parsley

Salt and pepper, to taste

1 Lightly grease the inside of the slow cooker with a teaspoon of oil. In large skillet, cook onion and mushrooms in the remaining oil until tender. Turn the heat off, place the spinach leaves over the mixture, and cover with a tight-fitting lid. Allow the spinach to steam under the lid for about 10 minutes, or until wilted.

2 In a large bowl, beat the eggs with the heavy cream until well mixed. Add the onion, mushroom, and spinach mixture, then the parsley, salt, and pepper, and stir until combined.

3 Pour the eggs and vegetables into the slow cooker, cover, and turn on Low. Cook for 1 to 2 hours, until eggs are thoroughly cooked. To test for doneness, insert a clean knife in the center. If it comes out clean, the dish is ready.

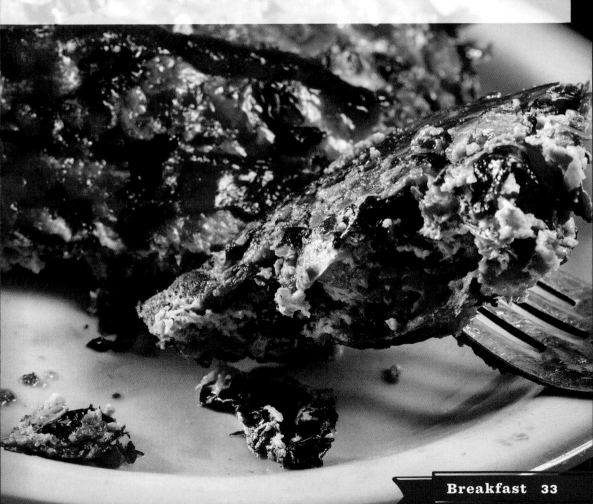

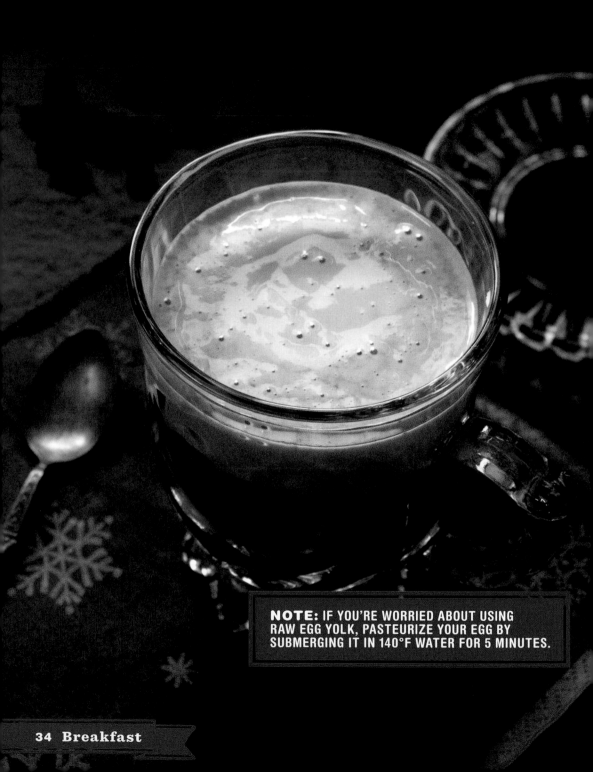

NOTE: IF YOU'RE WORRIED ABOUT USING RAW EGG YOLK, PASTEURIZE YOUR EGG BY SUBMERGING IT IN 140°F WATER FOR 5 MINUTES.

Vietnamese Egg Coffee

YIELD: 1 SERVING • PREP TIME: 5 MINUTES • COOK TIME: 5 MINUTES
NUTRITIONAL INFO: CALORIES: 97 • FAT: 8G • NET CARBS: 1G • PROTEIN: 3G

A staple in Vietnam, this rich, creamy, custard-like coffee not only fills you up, it also perks you up.

1 Blend together the egg yolk, cream, vanilla, and stevia for 3 to 4 minutes, until the mixture is a pale white color.

2 To serve, pour the ¼ cup of coffee into a mug, add the egg cream, and top with the remaining coffee.

INGREDIENTS

1 egg yolk

1 tablespoon heavy whipping cream

½ tablespoon vanilla extract

Stevia, to taste

¼ cup-plus 1 teaspoon freshly brewed Vietnamese coffee (or espresso)

Corned Beef and Cauliflower Hash

YIELD: 4 SERVINGS • PREP TIME: 10 MINUTES
COOK TIME: 45 MINUTES TO 1 HOUR 20 MINUTES
NUTRITIONAL INFO: CALORIES: 351 • FAT: 27G • NET CARBS: 4G • PROTEIN: 21G

For an even more filling breakfast, add eggs. Simply crack two eggs open over the hash mixture in the slow cooker before cooking. They will cook along with the hash. Just be sure to factor in an additional 20 to 30 minutes on Low or 15 to 30 on High.

INGREDIENTS

3 tablespoons butter

¼ cup onion, chopped fine

1 garlic clove, minced

2 cups cauliflower florets, diced

1 lb. corned beef, shredded

¼ cup chicken broth

Salt and pepper, to taste

1 In a skillet over medium-high heat, melt the butter. Add the onion and garlic and cook, stirring, until the onion is wilted, about 1 minute. Stir in the cauliflower pieces, warming them through. Remove the pan from the heat.

2 Coat the inside of the slow cooker with non-stick cooking spray and put the cauliflower mixture inside. Stir in the corned beef. Pour the chicken broth over everything.

3 Cover and cook on Low for 1 hour and 20 minutes or on High for about 45 to 60 minutes. Season with salt and pepper and serve hot.

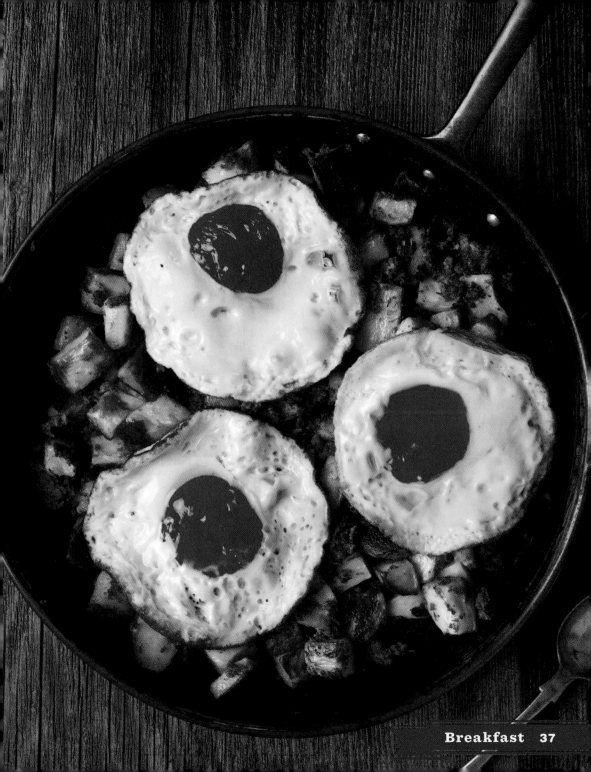

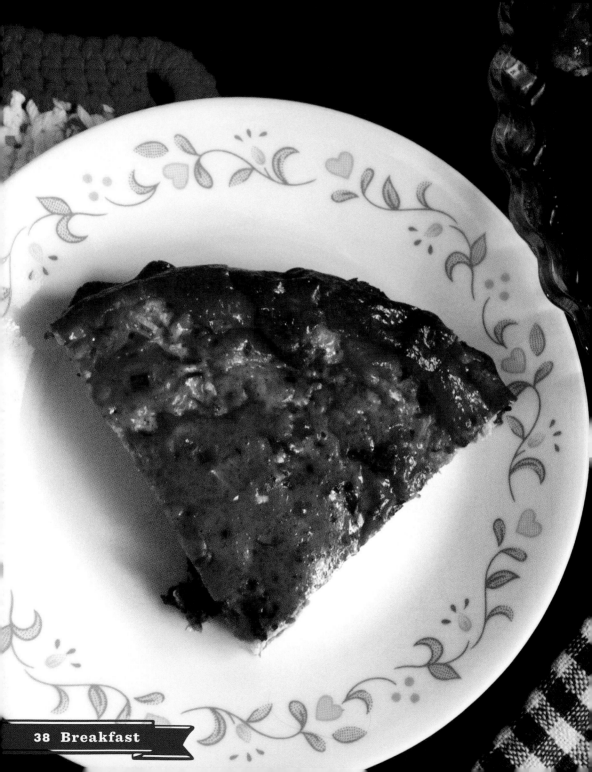

Crustless Quiche

YIELD: 2 SERVINGS • PREP TIME: 5 MINUTES • COOK TIME: 15 TO 20 MINUTES
NUTRITIONAL INFO: CALORIES: 561 • FAT: 44G • NET CARBS: 4G • PROTEIN: 34G

A quick and easy savory frittata-like quiche with chicken, olives, and sun-dried tomatoes.

1 Beat the eggs and cream in a bowl along with the salt, pepper, cayenne pepper, and paprika. Then, add in the cheese, chicken, chives, and sun-dried tomatoes and mix well.

2 Grease a baking dish or quiche dish with butter and pour in the mixture. Cook at 375°F for 15 to 20 minutes, until the quiche is cooked all the way through. Cut and serve.

INGREDIENTS

4 eggs

⅓ cup heavy whipping cream

¼ teaspoon salt

¼ teaspoon pepper

¼ teaspoon cayenne pepper

¼ teaspoon paprika

2¾ cups cheddar cheese

3½ cups cooked chicken breast, shredded

1 teaspoon chopped chives

¾ cup sun-dried tomatoes

1 tablespoon butter

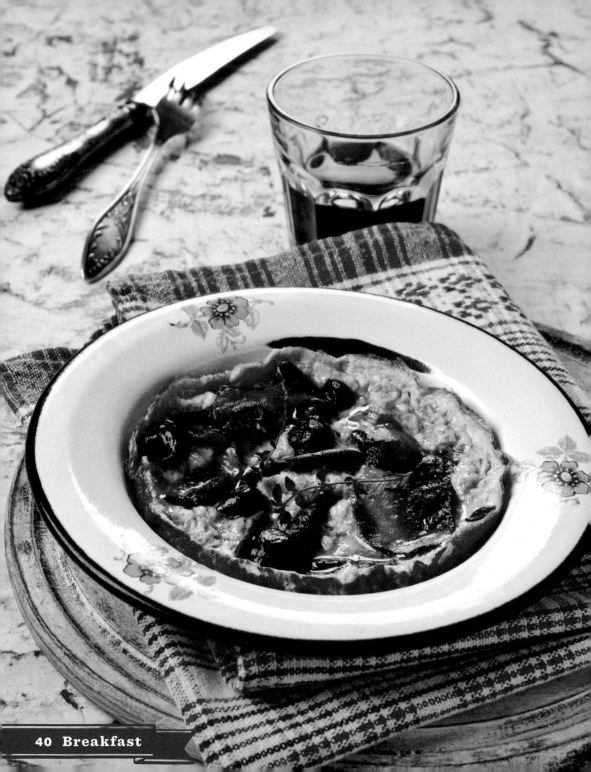

Mushroom and Swiss Cheese Frittata

YIELD: 4 SERVINGS • PREP TIME: 5 MINUTES • COOK TIME: 30 MINUTES
NUTRITIONAL INFO: CALORIES: 486 • FAT: 39G • NET CARBS: 8G • PROTEIN: 26G

The selection of mushrooms in grocery stores is getting bigger and bigger. You can use one kind of mushroom for this dish, or you can use several kinds together.

1 Melt the butter in the skillet over medium-high heat. Add the onion and cook, stirring, until translucent, about 3 minutes. Add the mushrooms, lower the heat slightly, and cook, stirring occasionally, until soft, 5 to 10 minutes. Drain the liquid from the pan. Season the mushrooms with the salt and pepper.

2 In a bowl, whisk the eggs with the heavy cream. Pour the egg mixture over the mushrooms. Sprinkle the cheese all around the top, and then sprinkle the parsley over everything.

3 Cover the skillet and let cook until set, about 10 minutes. Place the skillet in the oven under the broiler and "toast" the top until brown, about 2 minutes.

INGREDIENTS

3 tablespoons butter

½ cup onion, diced

1 lb. mushrooms, picked over and sliced or chopped

1 teaspoon salt

½ teaspoon pepper

8 eggs

½ cup heavy cream

1 cup Swiss cheese, shredded

⅓ cup fresh parsley, chopped

Spinach and Feta Frittata

YIELD: 4 SERVINGS • PREP TIME: 15 MINUTES • COOK TIME: 15 MINUTES
NUTRITIONAL INFO: CALORIES: 237 • FAT: 18G • NET CARBS: 3G • PROTEIN: 15G

This delicious breakfast gives a nod to Greek cuisine thanks to the feta cheese.

INGREDIENTS

6 eggs

2 tablespoons butter

¼ cup chopped red onion

1 garlic clove, minced

2 cups fresh spinach leaves, coarse stems removed, leaves roughly chopped

½ cup feta cheese

Salt and pepper, to taste

1 Preheat the broiler to low.

2 In a small bowl, beat the eggs with a whisk until combined.

3 Heat a skillet over medium-high heat. Melt the butter in the skillet and add the onions and garlic. Cook, while stirring, until the onions are translucent, about 3 minutes.

4 Add the spinach and stir so the leaves wilt. Sprinkle the feta over the mixture.

5 Pour the eggs over everything and shake the pan to evenly distribute them. Sprinkle with salt and pepper. Cover the skillet and let cook until set, about 10 minutes. Place the skillet in the oven under the broiler to toast the top, about 2 minutes.

6 Allow to stand for a couple of minutes and serve. Season with additional salt and pepper to taste.

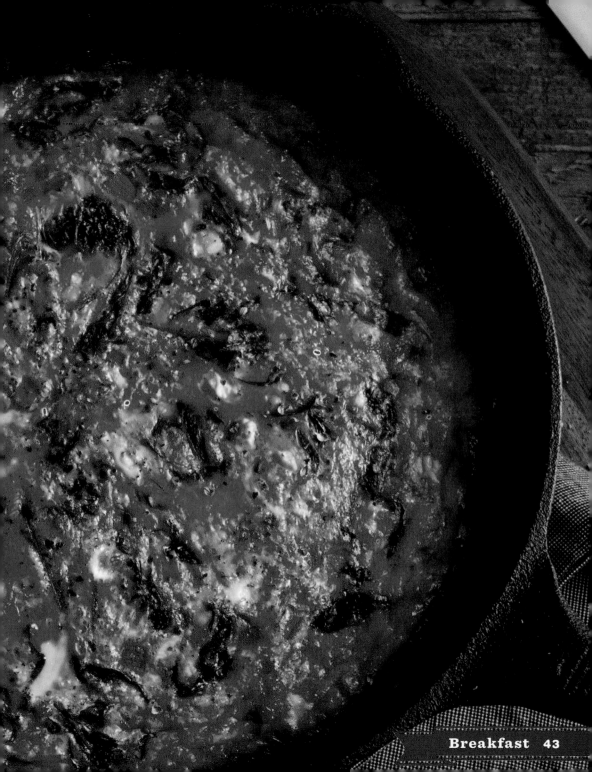

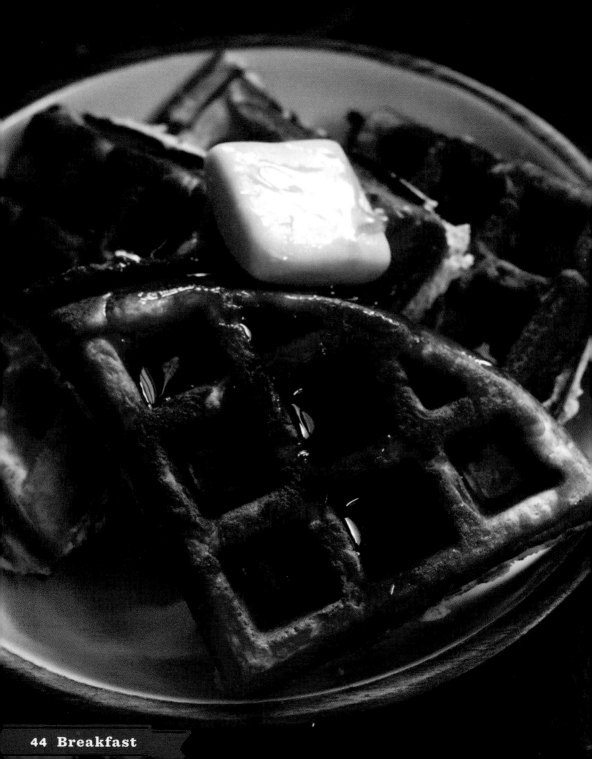

Coconut Flour Waffles

YIELD: 1 SERVING • PREP TIME: 5 MINUTES • COOK TIME: 10 MINUTES
NUTRITIONAL INFO: CALORIES: 620 • FAT: 51G • NET CARBS: 9G • PROTEIN: 19G

Coconut flour not only makes these waffles keto friendly, it also adds a whole new flavor dynamic to a breakfast favorite.

1 Microwave the mascarpone cheese for 30 seconds to soften it, then whisk together with the rest of the ingredients in a bowl. The batter should be thick but pourable. If the batter is too thick, add additional cream as needed to thin it out.

2 Heat your waffle iron and pour in the batter. Once cooked, remove and serve warm.

INGREDIENTS

2 tablespoons mascarpone cheese

¼ cup heavy whipping cream, plus 2 tablespoons to thin batter, if needed

4 tablespoons coconut flour

2 eggs

½ teaspoon baking powder

⅛ teaspoon salt

Stevia, to taste

Lemon and Peppercorn Poached Salmon

YIELD: 4 SERVINGS • PREP TIME: 15 MINUTES • COOK TIME: 2 TO 3 HOURS
NUTRITIONAL INFO: CALORIES: 643 • FAT: 44G • NET CARBS: 5G • PROTEIN: 51G

This is a really tasty and satisfying breakfast after a workout, especially an early morning run.

INGREDIENTS

6 cups water

½ cup onion, chopped

½ cup celery, chopped

4 sprigs parsley

½ cup lemon juice

8 whole black peppercorns

1 bay leaf

4 small salmon fillets
(approx. 8 oz. each)

4 tablespoons
salted butter

1 small lemon, sliced, for garnish

2 tablespoons fresh
parsley, chopped, for garnish

1 To prep the poaching liquid, combine water, onion, celery, parsley, lemon juice, peppercorns, and bay leaf in a saucepan over medium heat. Bring to a boil and simmer for 30 minutes. Strain and discard solids.

2 Take a large sheet of heavy-duty aluminum foil and place it inside the slow cooker so the sides extend beyond the top. Press it into place so it conforms with the inside of the cooker. Turn the cooker to High and preheat, still uncovered. Place the salmon over the foil in the slow cooker. Pour the hot poaching liquid over the salmon. Cover immediately and cook on High for 1 to 2 hours, until the flesh of the salmon is a light pink and firm.

3 Remove stoneware from slow cooker. Allow salmon to cool for 20 minutes before transferring to a platter and serving.

4 Melt the butter and pour a tablespoon over each fillet before serving.

5 Garnish with lemon slices and fresh parsley sprigs.

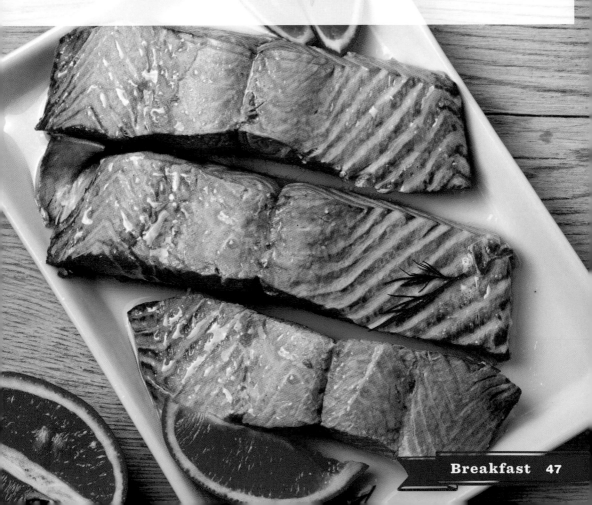

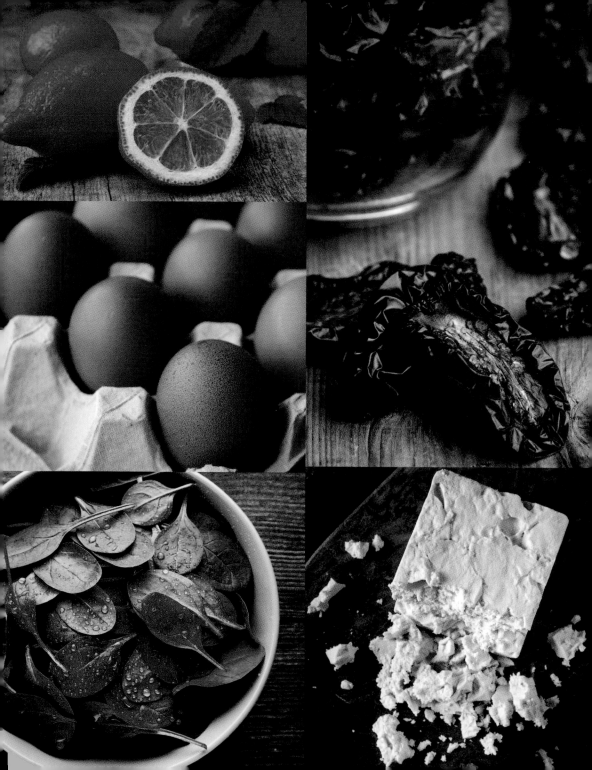

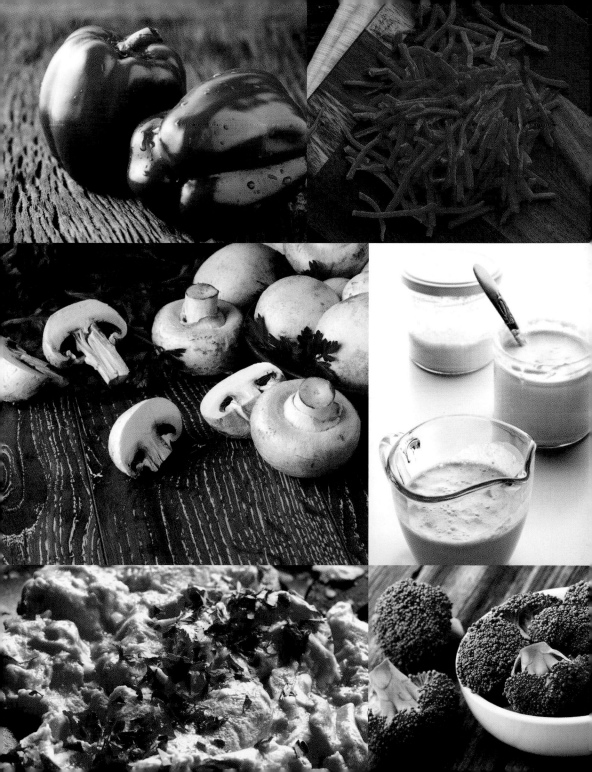

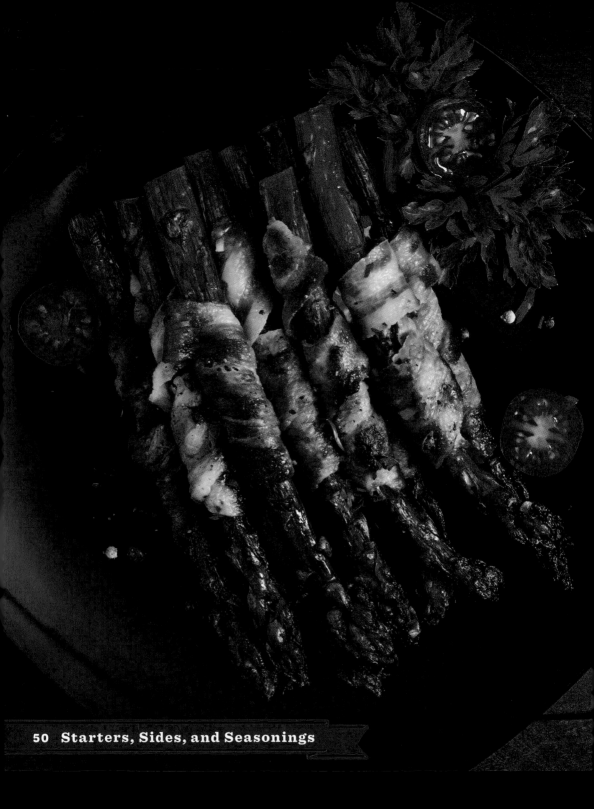

Starters, Sides, and Seasonings

On a diet, you hate feeling like you're missing out on good food, and on keto there's absolutely no reason to. Appetizers and sides are easily keto-customizable and a great way to build up to a stunning main course. A lot of these also work great as snacks and can be made in advance and saved for those times you're feeling a bit peckish between meals.

The sides and starters in this section strike a great balance between meat and veggies. Salads, full of vibrant greens and fresh vegetables; barbecue staples, skewers, sauces, and rubs for you to toss the choicest ingredients in—everything here is designed to excite your palate and keep keto interesting. There are also marinades that work great for meal prep—just marinate your favorite cuts of meat and freeze them so you can pull them out on a day when you're not in the mood to make an elaborate recipe.

Can you imagine anyone turning down Deviled Eggs with Bacon (page 52) or Stuffed White Mushrooms with Spanish Chorizo (page 88)?

Deviled Eggs with Bacon

YIELD: 6 SERVINGS • PREP TIME: 10 MINUTES • COOK TIME: 20 TO 25 MINUTES
NUTRITIONAL INFO: CALORIES: 514 • FAT: 50G • NET CARBS: 3G • PROTEIN: 2G

The recipe is very straightforward and is easy to adapt for a larger gathering so you can add any other flavors that come to mind!

INGREDIENTS

2 egg yolks, at room temperature

¼ medium lemon, juiced

1 cup light olive oil

10 large eggs

6 thick strips bacon

2 tablespoons Dijon mustard

2 tablespoons fresh parsley, finely chopped

Salt and pepper, to taste

1 teaspoon paprika (optional)

3 chives, finely chopped (optional)

1 In a small food processor, add the 2 egg yolks and the lemon juice and puree for 30 seconds. Very gradually, add in the light oil until you reach a thick, mayonnaise-like consistency. It is extremely important to make sure that you add the light oil slowly to the processor, if you go too quickly you will not reach the desired consistency.

2 Fill a medium saucepan with water. Carefully add the 10 eggs into the saucepan and then place the saucepan over medium heat. When the water reaches a boil, pull the eggs from the water and place under cool water. Let rest for a few minutes, and then peel back the shells.

3 Slice the eggs into halves. Using a fork, transfer the egg yolks from the eggs and place in a small bowl. Whisk in the mayonnaise-like mixture, the Dijon mustard, and parsley, and then season with salt and pepper. Set aside.

4 Place a medium frying pan over medium-high heat. Add the thick strips of bacon to the pan and cook until crispy, a few minutes on each side. If you would like to add a smoky flavor to the bacon, consider cooking the bacon on the grill. Transfer the bacon to a carving board and chop into bits. Whisk into the mixture.

5 Spoon the mixture from the small bowl back into the egg whites. If you would like, garnish with paprika and chopped chives and serve chilled.

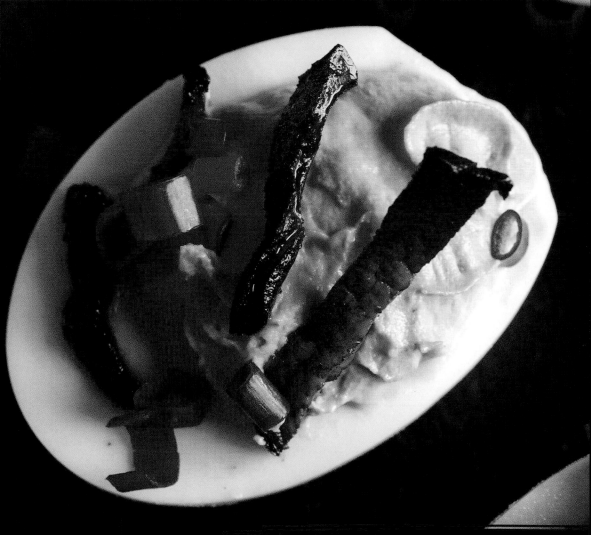

Butter Chicken Bites

YIELD: 5 SERVINGS • PREP TIME: 5 MINUTES • COOK TIME: 25 MINUTES
NUTRITIONAL INFO: CALORIES: 273 • FAT: 20G • NET CARBS: 2G • PROTEIN: 20G

A tangy and spicy tomato-and-cream sauce makes these bites perfect appetizers.

INGREDIENTS

17½ oz. boneless chicken thighs

Salt, to taste

2 tablespoons ghee

1 teaspoon tandoori masala

3¾ tablespoons butter

2 teaspoons ginger-garlic paste

½ teaspoon red chili powder

½ teaspoon turmeric

½ teaspoon garam masala

½ teaspoon coriander powder

½ teaspoon cumin powder

3⅓ tablespoons tomato puree

3⅓ tablespoons water

1 teaspoon dried fenugreek leaves

Stevia or sweetener of your choice, to taste

3⅓ tablespoons heavy whipping cream

Cilantro leaves, to taste, plus more for garnish

1 Cut the chicken into bite-sized pieces, then season with salt, 1 tablespoon ghee, and tandoori masala and set aside.

2 In a saucepan, heat the butter. Once the butter begins to foam, add the ginger-garlic paste along with the remaining dry spices. Cook until the butter has melted, then add in the tomato puree along with the water and the fenugreek leaves. Cover and cook for 5 minutes. Add in the sweetener and cook for another 5 minutes, then turn off the heat and add in cream and cilantro.

3 Heat up the remaining ghee in a frying pan and fry the chicken pieces until browned on all sides, then pour the sauce over the chicken and cook for about 5 minutes.

4 Once a sticky, glaze-like consistency is achieved, the chicken is ready. Garnish with additional cilantro and serve.

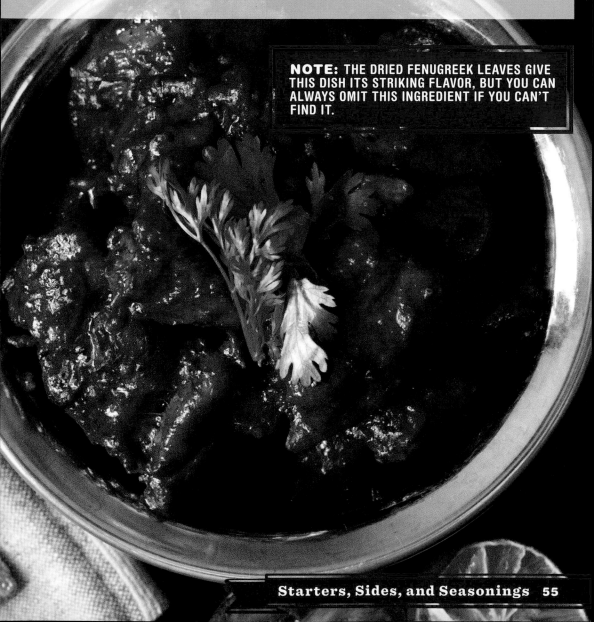

NOTE: THE DRIED FENUGREEK LEAVES GIVE THIS DISH ITS STRIKING FLAVOR, BUT YOU CAN ALWAYS OMIT THIS INGREDIENT IF YOU CAN'T FIND IT.

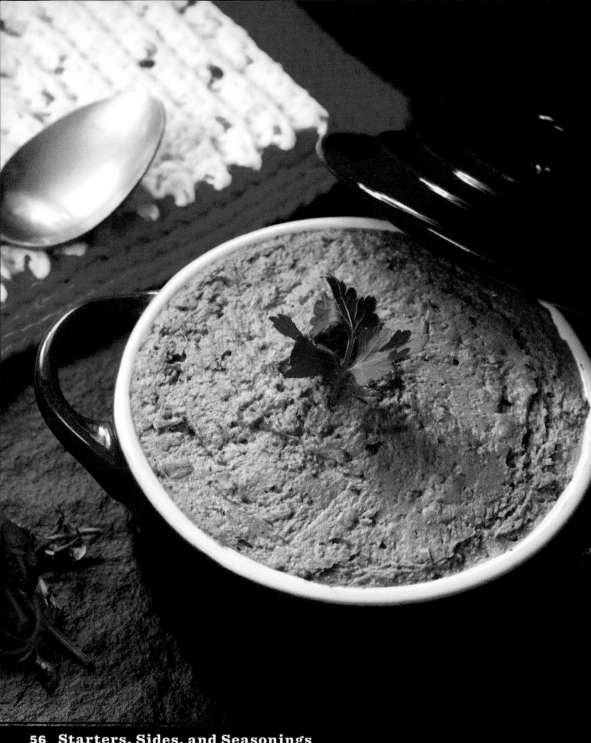

Chicken Liver Pâté

YIELD: 10 SERVINGS • PREP TIME: 5 MINUTES • COOK TIME: 10 MINUTES
NUTRITIONAL INFO: CALORIES: 70 • FAT: 6G • NET CARBS: 1G • PROTEIN: 4G

This decadent pâté makes a perfect spread for keto bread or crackers.

INGREDIENTS

- ½ tablespoon olive oil
- ¼ cup red onion, chopped
- 2 garlic cloves, chopped
- Salt and pepper, to taste
- ¼ teaspoon paprika
- 7 oz. chicken livers, chopped
- 1 teaspoon parsley
- 1 teaspoon thyme
- 3 tablespoons butter
- Olives, for garnish
- Keto bread or crackers, to serve

1 Heat the oil in a pan and sauté the onion and garlic, seasoning with salt, pepper, and paprika.

2 Once the onion turns translucent, add the livers and cook for 2 minutes. Season the livers with additional salt and pepper, add the herbs, and cook for 2 more minutes.

3 Once the livers are cooked, turn off the heat, add butter and mix until it's melted.

4 Blend the liver mixture in a food processor until it reaches the desired texture.

5 Transfer to a ramekin and refrigerate. Once chilled, garnish with olives and serve with keto bread or crackers.

Lemon Pepper Chicken Wings

YIELD: 7 SERVINGS (1 WING PER SERVING) • PREP TIME: 5 MINUTES • COOK TIME: 20 MINUTES
NUTRITIONAL INFO (FOR THE WINGS): CALORIES: 150 • FAT: 6G • NET CARBS: 1G • PROTEIN: 21G
NUTRITIONAL INFO (FOR THE DIP): CALORIES: 96 • FAT: 9G • NET CARBS: 1G • PROTEIN: 3G

Crispy, deep-fried wings are good on their own, but the delicious seasoning takes these to a whole new level.

INGREDIENTS

For the Wings

7 chicken wings

1 tablespoon olive oil

½ tablespoon lemon pepper seasoning

Bacon fat or lard, for deep frying

For the Dip

3¾ tablespoons heavy whipping cream

3¾ tablespoons cheese of choice (cheddar is recommended)

1 garlic clove, minced

Salt and pepper, to taste

Green part of a spring onion, sliced

1 Season the wings with the oil and lemon pepper seasoning.

2 In a Dutch oven, heat the bacon fat or lard and deep fry wings until golden brown, crispy, and cooked fully. This normally takes 5 minutes or so, depending on the size of the wing. Drain on paper towels.

3 To make the dip, combine the cream, cheese, garlic, salt, and pepper in a bowl and microwave for 30 seconds. Stir, then microwave for another 30 seconds. Stir until it's nice and smooth. If dip is too thick, add about ½ tablespoon of water.

4 Garnish the dip with the sliced spring onion and serve alongside the wings.

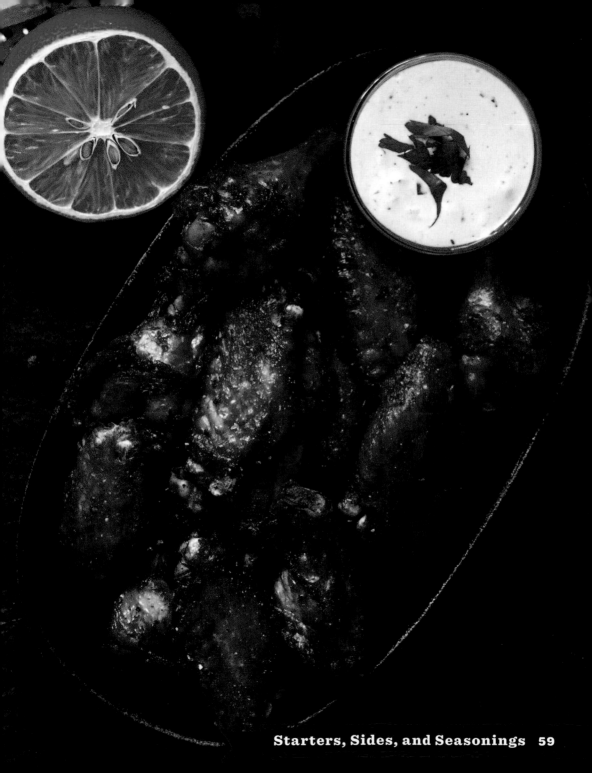

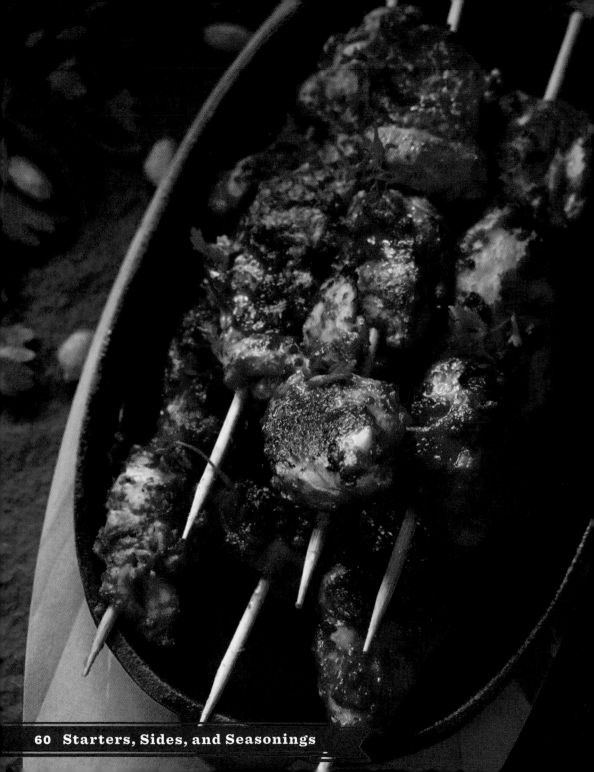

Peanut Butter Chicken Skewers

YIELD: 5 SERVINGS • PREP TIME: 15 MINUTES • COOK TIME: 15 MINUTES
NUTRITIONAL INFO: CALORIES: 144 • FAT: 6G • NET CARBS: 2G • PROTEIN: 18G

No matter where in the world you are, meat on a stick is always satisfying.

TOOLS

Wooden skewers

INGREDIENTS

1¼ tablespoons natural peanut butter with no added sugar

2 tablespoons coconut cream

2 teaspoons soy sauce

2 teaspoons fish sauce

3 teaspoons vinegar

2 teaspoons Sriracha

1 teaspoon ginger, grated

1 garlic clove, grated

½ teaspoon salt

½ teaspoon pepper

17½ oz. skinless and boneless chicken thighs, cut into bite-sized pieces

Cilantro leaves, for garnish

1 In a bowl, mix together all ingredients, except the chicken and cilantro, then add the chicken and stir until it is well coated.

2 Skewer the chicken to form the kebabs, then grill the skewers or bake in the oven at 425°F for 15 minutes.

3 Garnish with cilantro leaves and serve.

Smoky Buffalo Wings

YIELD: 6 SERVINGS • PREP TIME: ABOUT 2 HOURS • COOK TIME: 10 MINUTES
NUTRITIONAL INFO: CALORIES: 319 • FAT: 20G • NET CARBS: 7G • PROTEIN: 25G

Add smoke to these classic wings by adding a couple cups of soaked hickory or oak wood chips to the coals. This step is optional, but the resulting flavor is worth it.

INGREDIENTS

2 lbs. chicken wings, split

2 cups hickory or oak wood chips

2 tablespoons clarified butter

3 garlic cloves, minced

¼ teaspoon cayenne pepper

¼ teaspoon paprika

2 teaspoons Sriracha

1 head celery, stalks cut into 3-inch pieces, to serve

1 Place the chicken wings on a roasting pan and put in the refrigerator. Let rest for at least 2 hours so that the skin on the wings tightens, promoting a crisp wing.

2 One hour before grilling, add the wood chips into a bowl of water and let soak.

3 A half hour before grilling, prepare your gas or charcoal grill to high heat.

4 In a small saucepan, add the clarified butter over medium heat. Once hot, add the garlic and cook until golden—about 2 minutes. Next, mix in all of the remaining ingredients, minus the celery, and bring to a simmer over medium heat. Simmer for about 3 minutes and then remove from heat and place in a large bowl.

5 Remove the chicken wings from the refrigerator and toss with the buffalo sauce in the large bowl.

6 When the grill is ready, at about 450°F with the coals lightly covered with ash, scatter the wood chips over the coals or place them in a smoker box, and then place the chicken wings on the grill with a good amount of space between them. Cover the grill and cook for about 2 to 3 minutes on each side. Remove from grill when the skin is crispy.

7 Place on a large serving platter and serve warm alongside celery.

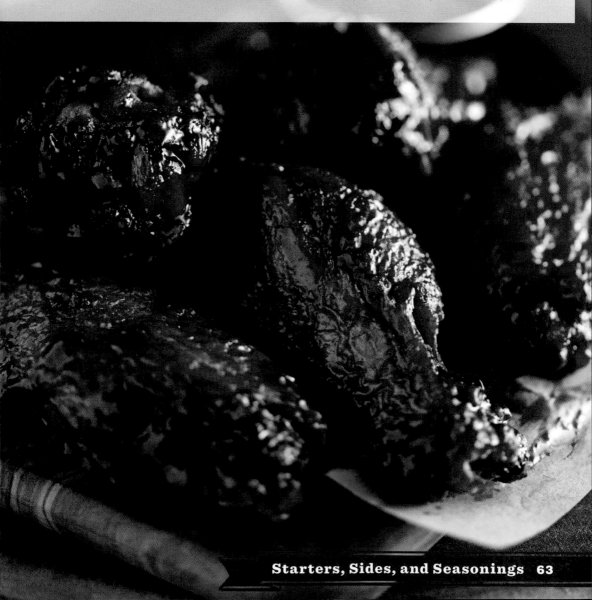

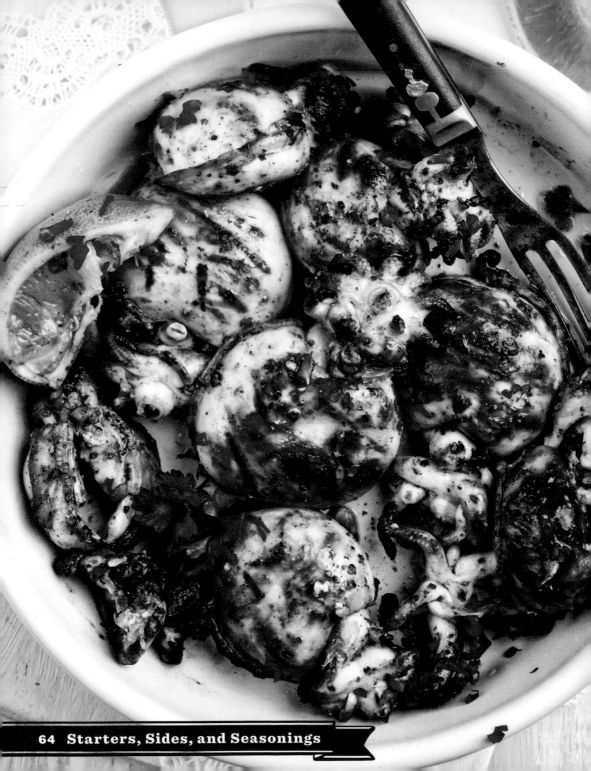

Grilled Garlic Calamari

YIELD: 6 SERVINGS • PREP TIME: 1 TO 2 HOURS • COOK TIME: ABOUT 10 MINUTES
NUTRITIONAL INFO: CALORIES: 224 • FAT: 11G • NET CARBS: 6G • PROTEIN: 24G

To hit your fat macros, add a tablespoon of butter to each serving.

INGREDIENTS

1 lemon, juiced

¼ cup extra virgin olive oil

2 garlic cloves, finely chopped

2 sprigs fresh oregano, leaves removed

Salt and pepper, to taste

2 lbs. fresh squid, tentacles separated from bodies

1 Combine the lemon juice, olive oil, garlic, and oregano in a large bowl. Season with salt and pepper. Add the squid to the bowl and let marinate for 1 to 2 hours.

2 Prepare your gas or charcoal grill to medium-high heat. Leave a cast-iron skillet on the grill while heating so that it develops a faint, smoky flavor.

3 When the grill is ready, at about 400°F with the coals lightly covered with ash, place the squid tentacles and rings in the skillet and cook until opaque, about 3 to 4 minutes. When finished, transfer the squid to a large carving board and let stand at room temperature for 5 minutes before serving.

Brussels Sprouts with Mustard Seasoning

YIELD: 4 SERVINGS • PREP TIME: 5 MINUTES • COOK TIME: 2 TO 4 HOURS
NUTRITIONAL INFO: CALORIES: 142 • FAT: 14G • NET CARBS: 2G • PROTEIN: 1G

Mustard adds a wonderful tanginess to this recipe, but you can substitute other spices to get different flavors. For spicier sprouts, add some cayenne pepper or hot sauce; for an Indian taste, add hints of curry or cumin.

INGREDIENTS

1 lb. Brussels sprouts

4 tablespoons extra virgin olive oil

1 teaspoon dry mustard

Salt, to taste

1 Wash and trim the Brussels sprouts, cutting off the coarsest part of the bottom and a layer or so of the leaves. Cut the sprouts in half and put them in the slow cooker.

2 In a measuring cup, mix the oil with the dry mustard. Pour over the Brussels sprouts. Cover and cook on Low for 3 to 4 hours or on High for 2 to 3 hours. Before serving, add a pinch of salt.

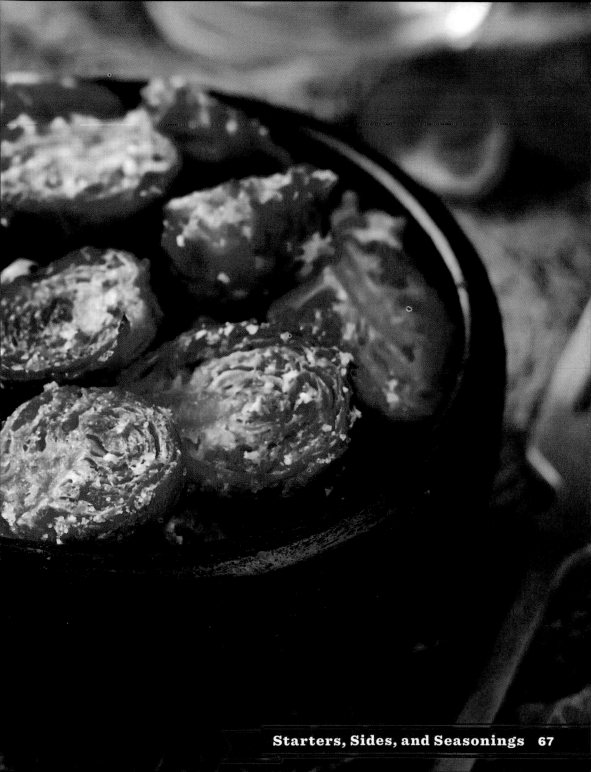

Cajun Eggplant

YIELD: 4 SERVINGS • PREP TIME: 5 MINUTES • COOK TIME: 10 MINUTES
NUTRITIONAL INFO: CALORIES: 162 • FAT: 15G • NET CARBS: 5G • PROTEIN: 2G

Serve this with one pound of skinless, boneless chicken breasts: grill over medium heat for 5 to 6 minutes, until thoroughly cooked through, and add a dollop of butter over each serving for extra flavor and fat.

INGREDIENTS

¼ cup extra virgin olive oil

2 tablespoons lime juice

1 tablespoon Cajun seasoning

2 small eggplants, cut into ½-inch slices (approx. 2 pounds total)

1 In a small bowl, mix together oil, lime juice, and Cajun seasoning. Brush this mixture over both sides of the eggplants and let them sit for about 5 minutes.

2 Preheat the grill to medium heat and then cook the slices until they become tender. This should take about 4 to 5 minutes per side. Remove from heat and serve.

Cajun-Spiced Grilled Green Beans

YIELD: 4 SERVINGS • PREP TIME: 5 MINUTES • COOK TIME: 20 MINUTES
NUTRITIONAL INFO: CALORIES: 140 • FAT: 12G • NET CARBS: 5G • PROTEIN: 2G

To add more protein, toss in some bacon. Just remove the packets after about 15 minutes and wrap the green beans in pieces of bacon that have been cut in half. Place them back in the foil packets or directly on the grill and cook until the beans are tender and the bacon is crisp.

INGREDIENTS

1 lb. green beans, trimmed

½ teaspoon Cajun seasoning

4 tablespoons butter

1 Prepare a large piece of foil to create a foil packet. Place the green beans on the foil and sprinkle the Cajun seasoning over them, along with butter. Fold the foil over the beans and crimp the edges to seal the packet tightly.

2 Preheat the grill to medium heat and place the packet on the grill seam side up. Cook for about 20 minutes, rotating the packet about 10 minutes in. Remove from heat when beans are tender and serve.

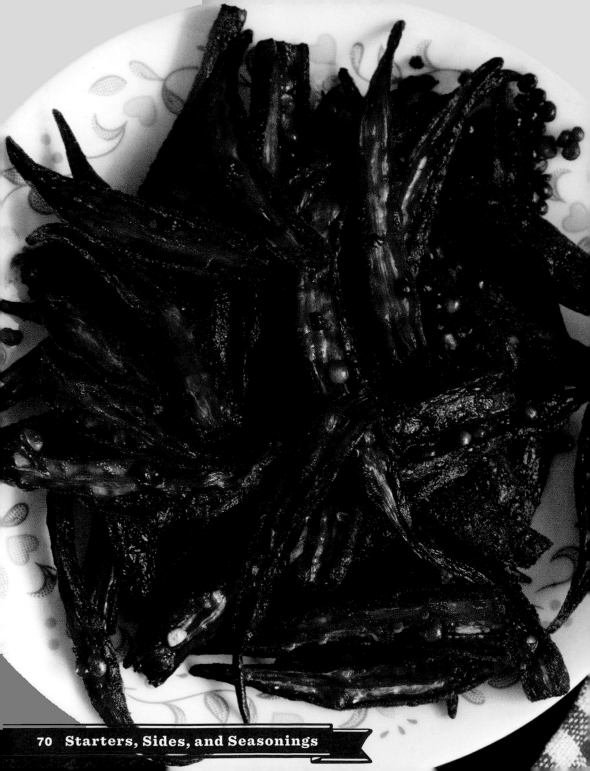

Crispy Fried Okra

YIELD: 2 SERVINGS • PREP TIME: 10 MINUTES • COOK TIME: 10 MINUTES
NUTRITIONAL INFO: CALORIES: 96 • FAT: 7G • NET CARBS: 5G • PROTEIN: 2G

A crunchy keto-safe snack of okra seasoned with spices.

1 Prepare the okra for frying, either by slicing and removing the seeds or leaving the seeds.

2 In a bowl, combine okra, oil, and seasonings.

3 Add the bacon fat or lard to a Dutch oven and deep fry the okra.

3 Once the okra is golden brown and crispy remove from oil and dry on paper towels. Serve immediately.

INGREDIENTS

2 cups okra

1 teaspoon olive oil

¼ teaspoon salt

¼ teaspoon paprika

¼ teaspoon cayenne pepper

Bacon fat or lard, for deep frying

Curried Kale Chips

YIELD: 2 SERVINGS • PREP TIME: 5 MINUTES • COOK TIME: 20 MINUTES
NUTRITIONAL INFO: CALORIES: 88 • FAT: 7G • NET CARBS: 3G • PROTEIN: 2G

Crunchy kale seasoned with curry powder—a perfect keto snack.

INGREDIENTS

3½ oz. kale

1 tablespoon olive oil

1 teaspoon curry powder

Salt, to taste

1 Wash and dry the kale, and then separate the leaves from the stalks and cut into small, bite-sized pieces.

2 Toss with the oil, curry powder, and salt and bake on a wire rack at 300°F for about 20 minutes, or until crispy.

3 Eat immediately. These chips lose their crispness over time.

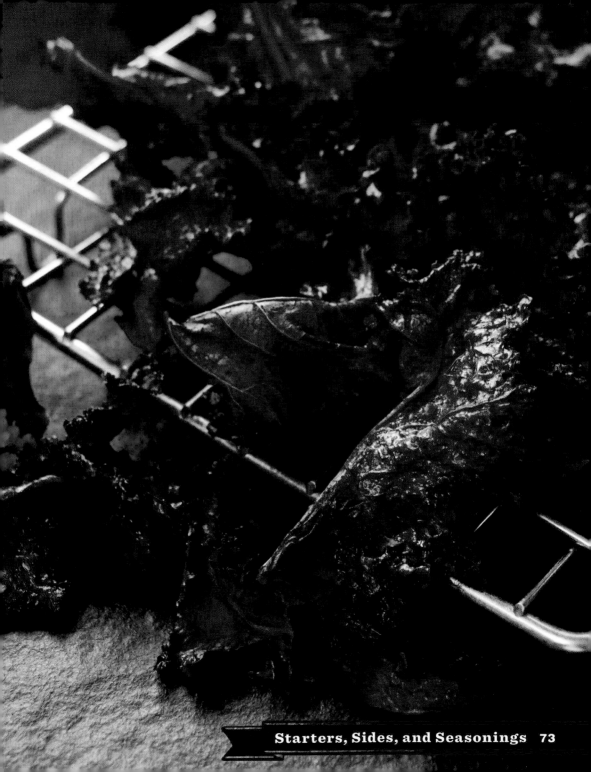

Mushroom and Bell Pepper Kebabs

YIELD: 4 SERVINGS • PREP TIME: 15 MINUTES • COOK TIME: 10 TO 15 MINUTES
NUTRITIONAL INFO: CALORIES: 137 • FAT: 11G • NET CARBS: 5G • PROTEIN: 3G

Mushroom kebabs are great because they soak up a marinade extremely well. The bell peppers ensure that this skewer is equal parts savory and refreshing.

TOOLS

4 wooden skewers

INGREDIENTS

½ lb. medium white mushrooms

½ cup bell pepper, cut into chunks

¼ cup onion, cut into chunks

¼ cup melted butter

½ teaspoon dill

½ teaspoon garlic salt

1 Thread mushrooms, pepper, and onion onto 4 skewers.

2 In a small bowl, combine butter, dill, and garlic salt. Brush this mixture over the skewered vegetables.

3 Preheat grill to medium-high heat and grill kebabs for 10 to 15 minutes, turning occasionally. Remove from heat and serve.

Grilled Cauliflower with Shredded Pepper Jack Cheese

YIELD: 4 SERVINGS • PREP TIME: 5 MINUTES • COOK TIME: ABOUT 10 MINUTES
NUTRITIONAL INFO: CALORIES: 231 • FAT: 19G • NET CARBS: 7G • PROTEIN: 7G

Steak isn't just for meat eaters. Try this vegetarian option featuring cauliflower fresh from the garden.

1 Begin by slicing the cauliflower lengthwise through the core into four pieces—these will become your "steaks." Preheat the grill to medium-high heat.

2 Mix the olive oil, lemon juice, garlic, red pepper flakes, salt, and pepper with a whisk.

3 Place the steaks into foil large enough to surround the steaks. Generously brush the mixture on both sides of the cauliflower. Seal the packet and place on the grill. Cook for about 8 minutes, or until tender. Flip the steaks about halfway through.

4 Once the cauliflower is slightly browned, remove from heat, sprinkle shredded pepper jack over the tops, and serve.

INGREDIENTS

1 large head cauliflower

¼ cup extra virgin olive oil

1 tablespoon lemon juice

2 garlic cloves, minced

Red pepper flakes, to taste

Salt and pepper, to taste

½ cup shredded pepper jack cheese

Grilled Lime Butter Broccoli

YIELD: 4 SERVINGS • PREP TIME: 5 MINUTES • COOK TIME: 10 MINUTES
NUTRITIONAL INFO: CALORIES: 309 • FAT: 26G • NET CARBS: 8G • PROTEIN: 4G

This is side gives off a soft flavor that will never overpower the main course. It's great alongside pork or poultry.

INGREDIENTS

6 tablespoons clarified butter

¼ small lime, juiced

2 garlic cloves, finely chopped

½ teaspoon finely chopped cilantro

Salt and pepper, to taste

2½ cups broccoli florets

2 tablespoons olive oil

1 Prepare your gas or charcoal grill to medium heat.

2 Combine the clarified butter, lime juice, garlic, and cilantro into a small saucepan over very low heat and stir occasionally. Season with salt and pepper.

3 When the grill is ready, about 400°F, brush the broccoli florets with oil and place on the grill. Cook until lightly charred, about 10 minutes, and then transfer to a medium bowl.

4 Remove the lime butter from the burner and then mix with the broccoli florets. Serve warm.

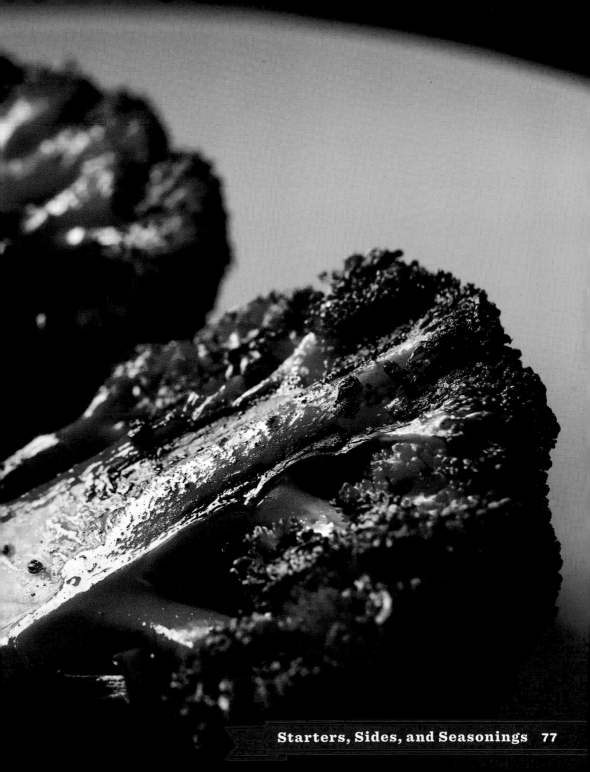

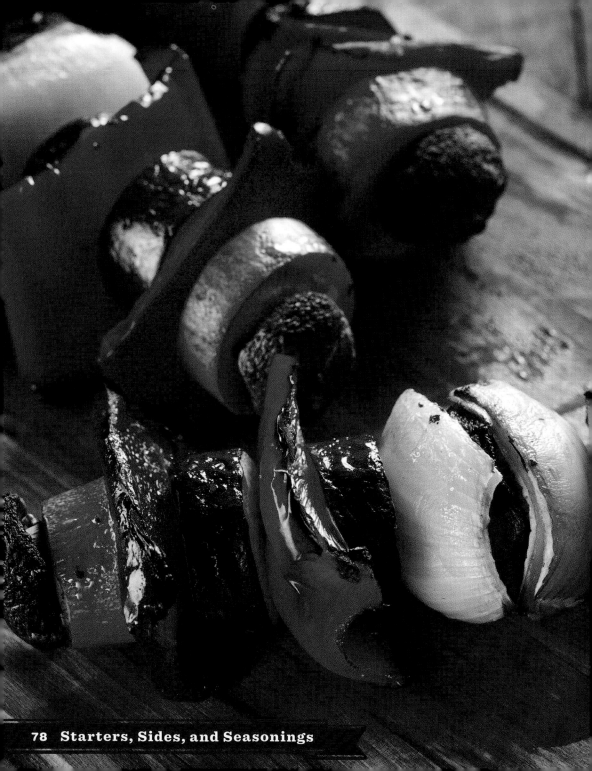

Grilled Vegetable Medley

SERVES: 6 SERVINGS • PREP TIME: 20 MINUTES • COOK TIME: 10 TO 12 MINUTES
NUTRITIONAL INFO: CALORIES: 188 • FAT: 17G • NET CARBS: 6G • PROTEIN: 2G

If you love mustard, increase the amount of Dijon you include in this recipe. Its sharp flavor profile pairs nicely with any fresh vegetable.

1 In a small bowl, combine the oil, red wine vinegar, dried oregano, Dijon, garlic, salt, and pepper and mix well.

2 Place the vegetables in a large, resealable bag and toss to coat with the dressing. Let this stand for about 15 minutes in the refrigerator.

3 Preheat the grill to medium heat and skewer the vegetables. Cook until they become tender, about 10 to 12 minutes. Remove from heat, top with the butter, and serve.

INGREDIENTS

¼ cup extra virgin olive oil

2 tablespoons red wine vinegar

½ teaspoon dried oregano

1 teaspoon Dijon mustard

1 garlic clove, minced

Salt and pepper, to taste

2 medium zucchini, cut into ¼-inch rounds

1 medium summer squash, cut into ¼-inch rounds

1 small red onion, cut into wedges

½ cup bell pepper, cut into 2-inch strips

4 to 5 small mushrooms

6 cherry tomatoes

4 tablespoons butter

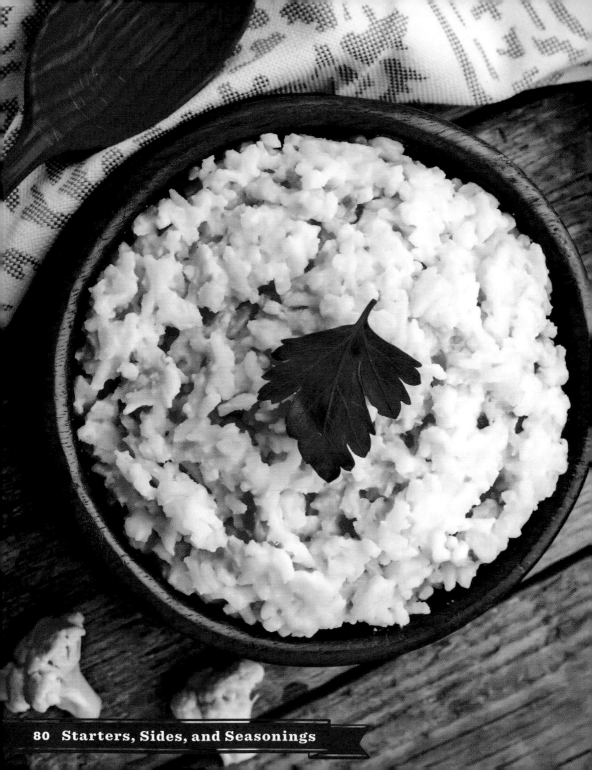

Riced Cauliflower

YIELD: 2 SERVINGS • PREP TIME: 5 MINUTES • COOK TIME: ABOUT 5 MINUTES
NUTRITIONAL INFO: CALORIES: 345 • FAT: 28G • NET CARBS: 11G • PROTEIN: 8G

This simple rice substitute gives you the texture of rice without the added carbs.

INGREDIENTS

1 large head cauliflower

4 tablespoons extra virgin olive oil

Salt and pepper, to taste

1 In a food processor, pulse the cauliflower until it becomes granular.

2 In a skillet over medium heat, heat oil and cook your cauliflower rice, covered, for 3 to 5 minutes. Sprinkle with salt and pepper to taste and serve.

Lemon Pepper Paneer

YIELD: 1 SERVING • PREP TIME: 5 MINUTES • TOTAL TIME: 10 MINUTES
NUTRITIONAL INFO: CALORIES: 324 • FAT: 28G • NET CARBS: 0G • PROTEIN: 16G

This fresh Indian farmer's cheese gets a bright kick when flavored with lemon and pepper.

INGREDIENTS

5 oz. paneer

1 tablespoon olive oil

½ teaspoon lemon pepper seasoning

2½ teaspoons butter

Parsley, for garnish

1 Cut the paneer into cubes, brush with olive oil on both sides, and coat with lemon pepper seasoning.

2 Heat the butter and any remaining oil in the skillet. Pan fry paneer until golden brown on both sides, flipping cubes once, approximately 10 minutes.

3 Garnish with parsley and serve.

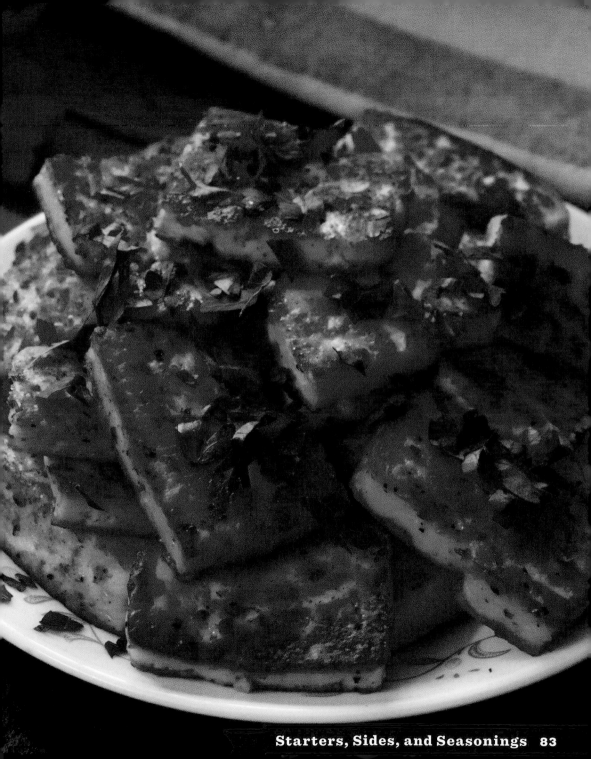

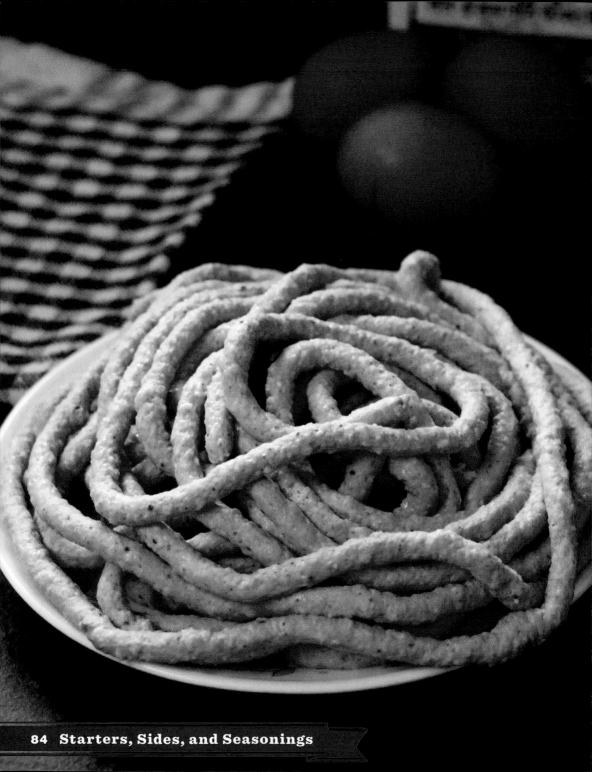

Chicken Noodles

YIELD: 2 SERVINGS • PREP TIME: 10 MINUTES • COOK TIME: ABOUT 1 MINUTE
NUTRITIONAL INFO: CALORIES: 301 • FAT: 7G • NET CARBS: 1G • PROTEIN: 52G

Use them as the base for your favorite dishes—like dandan noodles, spaghetti carbonara, and noodle soup. The variations are endless!

1 Blend all the ingredients in a food processor until you get a smooth paste.

2 Put the paste in a piping bag, or even a squeeze bottle. If using piping bag, cut the tip of the piping bag lower or higher depending on how thick you want the noodles to be.

3 Fill a saucepan with salted water and bring to a gentle simmer. Pipe in the noodles and then allow 20 to 25 seconds to cook. You'll know they're cooked when they rise to the surface. Remove with a slotted spoon.

INGREDIENTS

14 oz. chicken breasts

2 eggs

1 tablespoon psyllium husk powder

1 teaspoon Old Bay Seasoning

Sausage and Tomato-Stuffed Jalapeños

YIELD: 6 SERVINGS • PREP TIME: 10 MINUTES • COOK TIME: 25 MINUTES
NUTRITIONAL INFO: CALORIES: 257 • FAT: 19G • NET CARBS: 7G • PROTEIN: 7G

Grilled stuffed jalapeños are simple and quick to prepare. Although the jalapeños are considered a hot pepper, when you seed and grill them, their heat is toned down. For the sausage, if you are looking to save some time, pick up organic pork sausage (from a local butcher, if possible). It never fails!

INGREDIENTS

2 tablespoons olive oil

1 lb. pork sausage

2 garlic cloves, minced

¼ small red onion, minced

3 tablespoons red bell pepper, minced

8 cherry tomatoes, minced

12 jalapeño peppers, halved and seeded

Salt and pepper, to taste

1 Prepare your gas or charcoal grill to medium heat. Leave a cast-iron skillet on the grill while heating so that it develops a faint, smoky flavor.

2 When the grill is ready, at about 350°F to 400°F with the coals lightly covered with ash, heat the oil in the skillet and then add the pork sausage. Cook until the sausage is no longer pink and is evenly browned.

3 When the sausage is almost done, add the garlic and onion and cook until the onion is translucent, about 2 to 3 minutes. Stir in the red bell pepper and the cherry tomatoes and cook for another 2 minutes or so. Transfer the stuffing from the grill and let rest.

4 Arrange the halves of the jalapeño peppers evenly on a baking sheet. Using a spoon, add the stuffing into the cavities of the peppers. Transfer to the grill and cook, with the grill covered, for about 20 minutes until lightly browned. Remove from the grill, season with salt and pepper, and serve immediately.

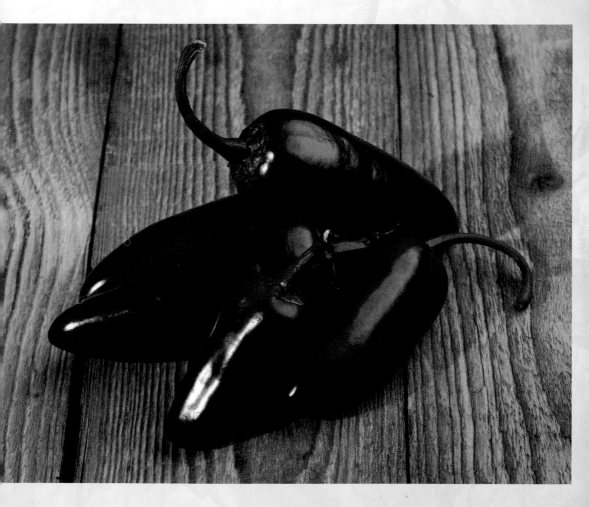

Stuffed White Mushrooms with Spanish Chorizo

YIELD: 6 SERVINGS • PREP TIME: 10 MINUTES • COOK TIME: 25 MINUTES
NUTRITIONAL INFO: CALORIES: 257 • FAT: 19G • NET CARBS: 7G • PROTEIN: 7G

Macros will vary depending on the brand and size of the chorizo used. Add some cheddar cheese to up the fat macros of the dish and also for a deliciously cheesy stuffed mushroom.

INGREDIENTS

1 Spanish chorizo, casing removed (approx. 4 oz.)

14 white mushrooms, stemmed

¼ cup plus 2 tablespoons extra virgin olive oil

¼ cup white onion, finely chopped

¼ cup chicken broth

1 small bunch parsley, finely chopped

Salt and pepper, to taste

1 Prepare your gas or charcoal grill to medium heat. Leave a cast-iron skillet on the grill while heating so that it develops a faint, smoky flavor.

2 While waiting, place the chorizo into a food processor and puree into a thick paste. Remove and set aside.

3 When the grill is ready, at about 350°F to 400°F with the coals lightly covered with ash, brush the mushroom caps with the 2 tablespoons of oil. Next, place the mushroom tops on the grill and cook for about 2 minutes until the tops have browned. Remove from grill and place on a baking sheet.

4 Next, add the remaining ¼ cup of oil to the cast-iron skillet, followed by the onion. Cook until the onion is translucent, about 2 minutes, and then stir in the pureed chorizo. Continue to cook until the chorizo is lightly browned, about 3 minutes, and then add in the chicken broth and parsley. Cook for only a minute or so longer, and then remove from heat.

5 Using a spoon, add the chorizo mixture into the mushroom caps. Move the baking sheet to a cool side of the grill and cook for about 15 minutes until the chorizo has browned. Remove from the grill, season with salt and pepper, and serve hot.

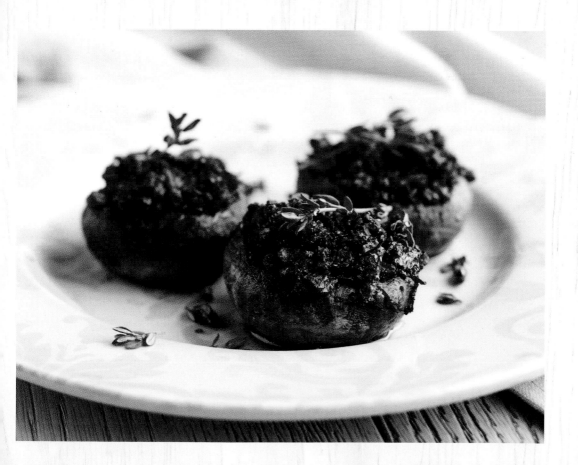

Arugula and Green Bean Side Salad

YIELD: 8 SERVINGS • PREP TIME: 10 MINUTES • COOK TIME: 20 MINUTES
NUTRITIONAL INFO: CALORIES: 86 • FAT: 8G • NET CARBS: 3G • PROTEIN: 2G

For a more filling salad, prepare $1^{1}/_{4}$ pounds of skirt steak by seasoning with salt and pepper. Grill this for 5 minutes per side, or until it reaches desired doneness. Serve slices of the steak over the salad.

INGREDIENTS

3 cups fresh green beans

6 tablespoons extra virgin olive oil

Salt and pepper, to taste

4 cups arugula

2 tablespoons balsamic vinegar

1 red bell pepper, chopped

1 Clean and trim green beans, then coat them with 2 tablespoons of the oil. Add salt and pepper to taste.

2 Preheat the grill to medium heat and coat the grates with 3 tablespoons of the oil. Spread the beans over the grate. Cover and cook for 15 to 20 minutes, making sure to rotate.

3 Once the beans are crispy and cooked through, remove them and toss with arugula, vinegar, bell pepper, and the remaining oil.

Asparagus Salad with Parmesan and Almonds

YIELD: 4 SERVINGS • PREP TIME: 5 MINUTES • COOK TIME: 15 TO 20 MINUTES
NUTRITIONAL INFO: CALORIES: 106 • FAT: 11G • NET CARBS: 3G • PROTEIN: 1G

This salad is asparagus-centric, but it's just as easy to substitute the spears for any other vegetable you prefer.

1 Preheat grill to low heat. In a bowl, combine oil, lemon juice, and asparagus, and toss to coat the asparagus.

2 Grill the asparagus spears for about 5 minutes, making sure to turn while cooking. Remove from heat once tender.

3 In a large serving bowl, combine the spring greens, Parmesan cheese, almond slices, cherry tomatoes, salt, and pepper.

4 Slice the asparagus into bite-sized pieces and add them to the salad with the lemon juice and oil. Toss the salad and serve.

INGREDIENTS

¼ cup extra virgin olive oil

¼ cup lemon juice

1 bunch asparagus spears

6 cups spring greens salad mix

2 tablespoons Parmesan cheese, grated

1 tablespoon almond slices

1 cup cherry tomatoes

Salt and pepper, to taste

Bacon and Frisée Salad with Hard-Boiled Eggs

YIELD: 6 SERVINGS • PREP TIME: 10 MINUTES • COOK TIME: 10 TO 15 MINUTES
NUTRITIONAL INFO: CALORIES: 152 • FAT: 12G • NET CARBS: 3G • PROTEIN: 7G

This salad is filling enough to be served as the main course.

1 One hour before grilling, soak the wood chips in water.

2 Next, place a large cast-iron skillet on your gas or charcoal grill and prepare to medium heat. Leave the grill covered while heating, as it will add a faint smoky flavor to the skillet.

3 While waiting, rinse the frisée and dry thoroughly. Place the frisée in a medium bowl and store it in the refrigerator.

4 Next, fill a medium saucepan with water and place over medium-heat. Bring to a boil and then add the eggs and remove from heat. Cover the saucepan and let the eggs rest in the hot water for about 10 to 14 minutes. Remove from water and let cool in the refrigerator.

5 When the grill is ready, at about 400°F with the coals lightly covered with ash, throw the wood chips over the

INGREDIENTS

1 cup maple wood chips

1 lb. frisée

3 large eggs

8 thick strips bacon

2 tablespoons white wine vinegar

2 tablespoons red wine vinegar

1 teaspoon Dijon mustard

2 tablespoons olive oil

Salt and pepper, to taste

coals or place them in a smoker box and cover the grill. When the grill is smoking, add the bacon into the cast-iron skillet, close the grill lid, and cook until crispy, about 4 minutes. Transfer to a plate covered with paper towels and chop when cool enough to handle.

6 In a small bowl, whisk together the white wine vinegar, red wine vinegar, Dijon mustard, and oil and then set aside.

7 Remove the eggs from the refrigerator and then peel off their shells. Slice the eggs in half and add over the frisée salad. Drizzle the vinaigrette onto the frisée and then top with the bacon bits. Season the eggs with the salt and pepper and then serve the salad immediately.

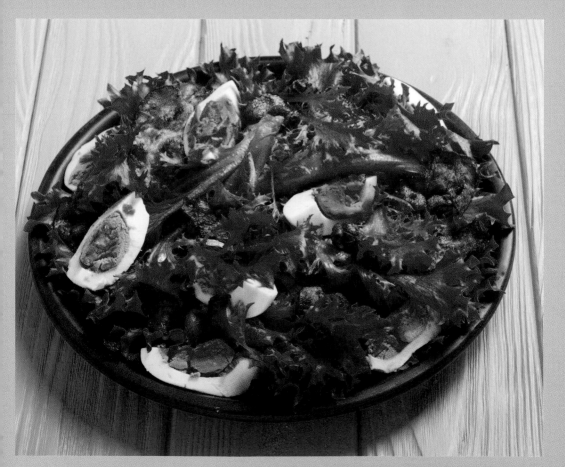

Caesar Salad

YIELD: 6 SERVINGS • PREP TIME: 20 MINUTES
NUTRITIONAL INFO: CALORIES: 205 • FAT: 20G • NET CARBS: 3G • PROTEIN: 4G

Top this salad with grilled chicken or smoked bacon for added protein.

INGREDIENTS

3 heads romaine lettuce

2 garlic cloves, minced

½ small lemon, juiced

1 large egg

4 anchovy fillets

1 teaspoon Dijon mustard

½ cup extra virgin olive oil

Salt and pepper, to taste

1 Rinse the heads of romaine lettuce and then dry thoroughly. Place in refrigerator and set aside.

2 In a small bowl, whisk the minced garlic, lemon juice, and egg until blended. Whisk in the anchovy fillets and Dijon mustard until the anchovies have been completely incorporated into the dressing.

3 Gradually whisk in the oil and then season with salt and pepper. Place the dressing in the refrigerator for about 15 minutes and then pour over the chilled romaine lettuce. Serve immediately.

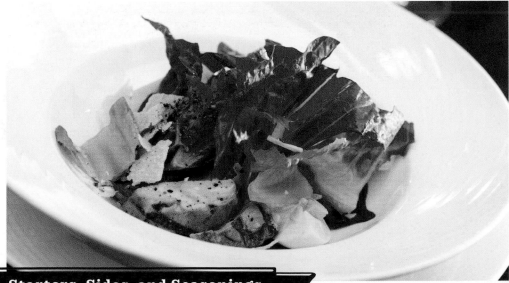

Caprese Salad

YIELD: 1 SERVING • PREP TIME: 5 MINUTES
NUTRITIONAL INFO: CALORIES: 444 • FAT: 38G • NET CARBS: 4G • PROTEIN: 22G

This keto spin on the classic Italian salad is easy and tasty.

INGREDIENTS

1 tomato, chopped

3½ oz. fresh buffalo mozzarella, chopped

1 teaspoon pine nuts

1 tablespoon Basil Pesto (see page 105)

1 Combine all ingredients in bowl, mix well, and serve.

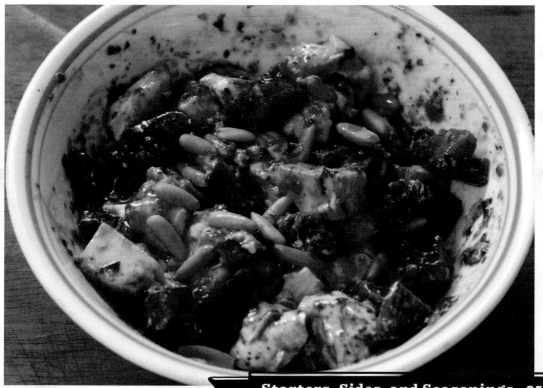

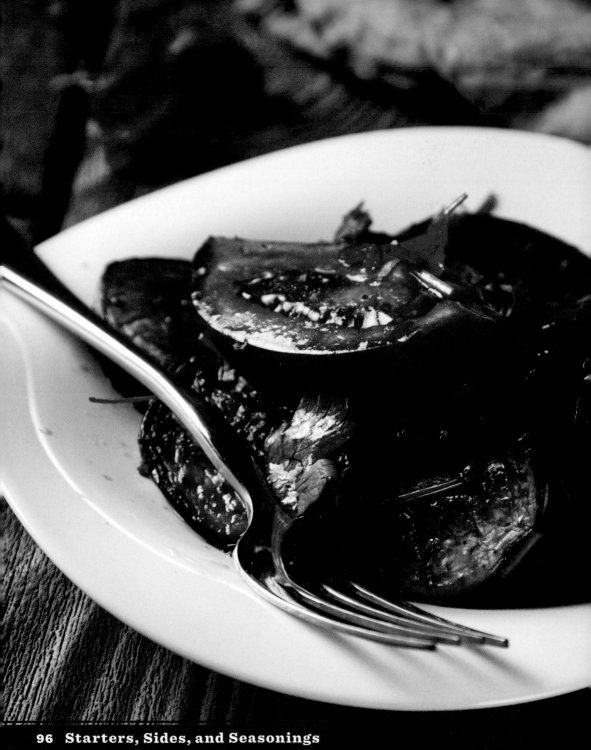

Grilled Eggplant Salad

YIELD: 3 SERVINGS • PREP TIME: 5 MINUTES • COOK TIME: 15 MINUTES
NUTRITIONAL INFO: CALORIES: 169 • FAT: 14G • NET CARBS: 6G • PROTEIN: 2G

If you are not a fan of eggplant try substituting your favorite squash instead.

1 Preheat grill to medium-high heat. Prick the eggplant with a fork, place on the grill, and cook for about 15 minutes with the grill covered. Cook until the skin is soft, turning eggplant occasionally. Remove from heat and let cool.

2 Once the eggplant is cool, scoop out the insides and chop. Place them in a bowl and toss with tomatoes, vinegar, oregano, garlic, and salt. Add in the oil, parsley, and pepper. Mix together and serve.

INGREDIENTS

1 large eggplant

1 medium tomato, chopped

1½ teaspoons red wine vinegar

½ teaspoon oregano

2 garlic cloves, diced

Salt, to taste

3 tablespoons extra virgin olive oil

3 tablespoons parsley, chopped

Black pepper, to taste

Grilled Portobello and Mozzarella Salad

YIELD: 4 SERVINGS • PREP TIME: 5 MINUTES • COOK TIME: ABOUT 10 MINUTES
NUTRITIONAL INFO: CALORIES: 160 • FAT: 11G • NET CARBS: 6G • PROTEIN: 8G

A grill can improve any salad and no recipe exemplifies that concept better than one with grilled portobello mushrooms. Enjoy this Italian-style salad in any season.

INGREDIENTS

7 grape tomatoes, halved

½ cup fresh mozzarella, cubed

6 fresh basil leaves, torn

4 tablespoons extra virgin olive oil

2 garlic cloves, minced

Salt and pepper, to taste

4 large portobello mushrooms

2 cups salad greens

1 In a small bowl, mix together tomatoes, mozzarella, basil leaves, half of the oil, garlic, salt, and pepper. Set the mixture aside.

2 Remove the stems and gills from mushrooms and lightly brush with the remaining oil.

3 Preheat the grill to medium-high heat. Grill the mushrooms with the grill covered for 6 to 8 minutes, until tender.

4 Remove from heat and dice the mushrooms.

5 In a large bowl toss the tomato mixture, salad greens, and diced mushrooms, and serve.

House Salad with Kalamata Olives and Pepperoncini

YIELD: 6 SERVINGS • PREP TIME: 20 MINUTES
NUTRITIONAL INFO: CALORIES: 308 • FAT: 30G • NET CARBS: 6G • PROTEIN: 3G

This basic salad is a good complement to a large steak or pork chop.

INGREDIENTS

3 heads romaine lettuce

1 small red onion, sliced into ¼-inch rings

10 Kalamata olives

10 green olives

4 plum tomatoes, stemmed and quartered

6 pepperoncini peppers

2 garlic cloves, minced

¼ cup red wine vinegar

¾ cup extra virgin olive oil

Salt and pepper, to taste

1 Rinse the heads of romaine lettuce and dry them thoroughly. In a medium bowl, combine the lettuce, red onion, Kalamata olives, green olives, tomatoes, and pepperoncini peppers and then set in the refrigerator.

2 In a small jar, whisk together the minced garlic, red wine vinegar, and oil, and then season with salt and pepper. Chill in refrigerator for 15 minutes.

3 Remove the salad and the vinaigrette from the refrigerator and mix together. Serve immediately.

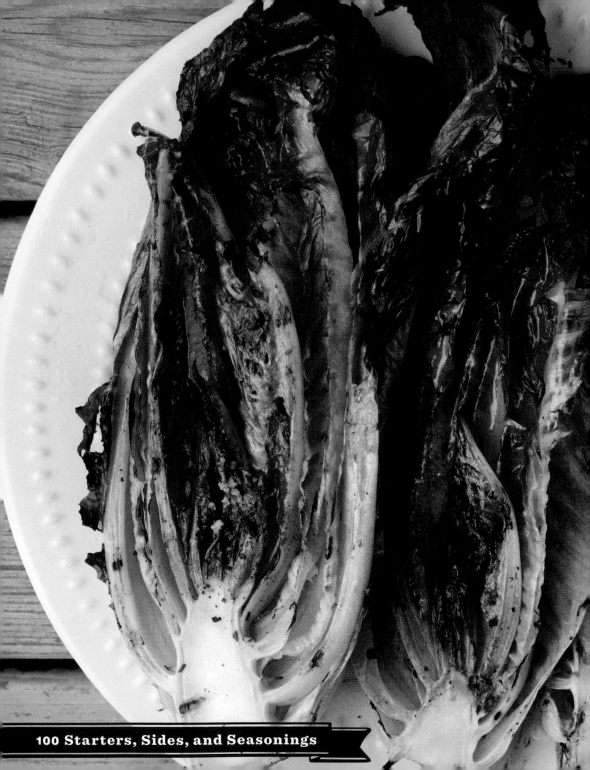

Grilled Romaine Wedge Salad

YIELD: 4 SERVINGS • PREP TIME: 10 MINUTES • COOK TIME: 5 MINUTES
NUTRITIONAL INFO: CALORIES: 99 • FAT: 8G • NET CARBS: 3G • PROTEIN: 3G

Grilled romaine may feel a bit uninspired, but the common leafy green provides a nice crunch that is lovely when paired with the steak seasoning.

1 Toss romaine lettuce with oil and season with steak seasoning.

2 Preheat the grill for medium heat. Oil the grates lightly to prevent sticking. Place the lettuce directly on the grill cut side down and cook for about 5 minutes. The lettuce is done cooking when it becomes slightly wilted and lightly charred.

3 Remove from heat, drizzle with lemon juice, and sprinkle Parmesan cheese on top. Serve and enjoy.

INGREDIENTS

1 head romaine lettuce, cut in half lengthwise

2 tablespoons extra virgin olive oil, plus more for grill

1 tablespoon steak seasoning

2 tablespoons lemon juice

2 tablespoons Parmesan cheese, for sprinkling

Pesto & Feta Salad with Calamari and Chorizo

YIELD: 1 SERVING • PREP TIME: 10 MINUTES • COOK TIME: 10 MINUTES
NUTRITIONAL INFO: CALORIES: 694 • FAT: 59G • NET CARBS: 4G • PROTEIN: 33G

Crispy chorizo and grilled calamari add wonderful depth to this salad.

INGREDIENTS

For the Dressing
1¼ oz. feta cheese
4 tablespoons olive oil
Salt and pepper, to taste

For the Salad
1 tablespoon olive oil
1 tablespoon butter
3 garlic cloves, chopped
3½ oz. calamari, with the rings cut into strips
1 tablespoon Basil Pesto (see page 105)
2 teaspoons Parmesan cheese, grated
1¼ oz. chorizo sausage, crumbled
1¾ oz. mixed lettuce

1 Mix all the dressing ingredients in a blender until the mixture has a rich, creamy, mayo-like texture. Add water to thin, if desired.

2 To make the salad, heat oil and butter in a pan and, once foaming, add the garlic.

3 Once the garlic starts to brown, add the calamari, followed by the Basil Pesto and half of the Parmesan cheese. Mix well.

4 In a separate pan, fry the chorizo until it releases its oils and crisps up.

5 Combine the lettuce and ⅓ of the dressing per serving, then top with the calamari.

6 Garnish with the remaining Parmesan and the fried chorizo and serve.

Tarragon-Shallot Vinaigrette Arugula Salad

YIELD: 6 SERVINGS • PREP TIME: 5 MINUTES
NUTRITIONAL INFO: CALORIES: 184 • FAT: 19G • NET CARBS: 3G • PROTEIN: 2G

This delicious, low-sugar salad is quick and easy to make, and the tarragon-shallot vinaigrette is so good, you'll forget you're eating healthy.

1 Rinse the arugula and then dry thoroughly. Place in refrigerator and set aside.

2 In a small bowl, whisk together the shallot, tarragon, lemon juice, and Dijon mustard, and then slowly add in the oil and red wine vinegar.

3 Season with salt and pepper, and then pour over the arugula. Serve immediately.

INGREDIENTS

1 lb. arugula lettuce, stemmed

1 shallot, minced

5 sprigs tarragon, minced

¼ small lemon, juiced

1 teaspoon Dijon mustard

½ cup extra virgin olive oil

3 tablespoons red wine vinegar

Salt and pepper, to taste

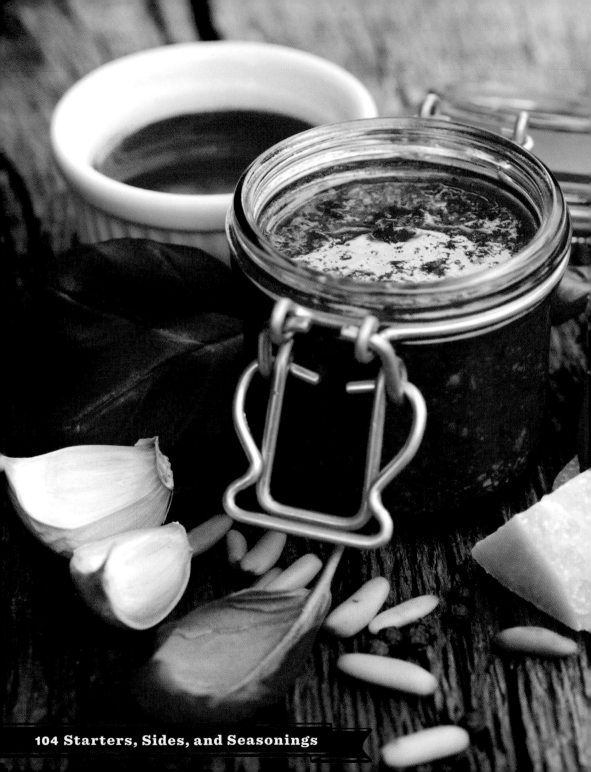

Basil Pesto

YIELD: 12 SERVINGS • PREP TIME: 5 MINUTES
NUTRITIONAL INFO: CALORIES: 142 • FAT: 16G • NET CARBS: 0G • PROTEIN: 2G

A keto essential that packs a wallop of flavor, whether as a marinade or a sauce.

1 In a dry pan, toast the pine nuts for 2 to 3 minutes.

2 Place the toasted pine nuts and remaining ingredients in a blender or food processor. Blend until mixture forms a smooth paste.

3 Use immediately or store in the refrigerator in a closed container.

INGREDIENTS

1½ tablespoons pine nuts

2¼ tablespoons Parmesan cheese, grated

1 garlic clove

2¼ tablespoons parsley

3¾ tablespoons basil

¾ cup extra virgin olive oil

Fresh lemon juice, to taste

Salt, to taste

Pasta Sauce with Meat

YIELD: 10 SERVINGS • PREP TIME: 10 MINUTES • COOK TIME: 2 TO 6 HOURS

NUTRITIONAL INFO: CALORIES: 209 • FAT: 13G • NET CARBS: 4G • PROTEIN: 19G

While you can't eat regular pasta on a low-carb diet, you can make a delightful bowl of spaghetti squash on which to serve this sauce. You can also slice zucchini with a mandoline to make "noodles." When you have been on the low-carb diet for a while, you can experiment with low-carb pastas, but they must be eaten only on occasion.

INGREDIENTS

2 tablespoons extra virgin olive oil

2 tablespoons butter

1 medium onion, chopped fine

1 green bell pepper, seeds and ribs removed, chopped fine

10 button mushrooms, rinsed and sliced thick

1 lb. ground beef

1 lb. ground turkey

2 (14.5 oz. each) cans of diced tomatoes, with their juices

3 garlic cloves, minced

2 teaspoons dried oregano

1 tablespoon dried basil

1 teaspoon red pepper flakes

Salt and pepper, to taste

1 In a large skillet over medium-high heat, add the oil, butter, onion, bell pepper, and mushrooms. Cook, while stirring, for about 3 minutes, and put in the bottom of the slow cooker.

2 In the same skillet, brown the ground meats together over medium heat, being careful not to cook too long. The meat should be slightly pink. Put it in the slow cooker on top of the vegetables.

3 Add the tomatoes and their juices, garlic, oregano, basil, and red pepper flakes. Stir to combine. Cover and cook on Low for 4 to 6 hours or on High for about 2 hours. Season with salt and pepper before serving.

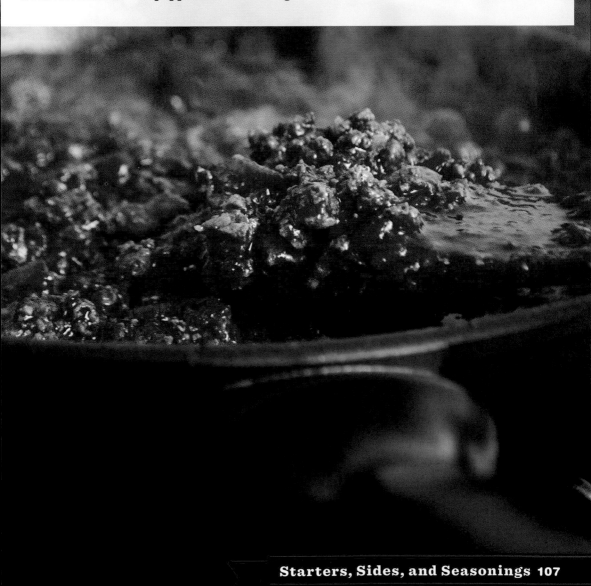

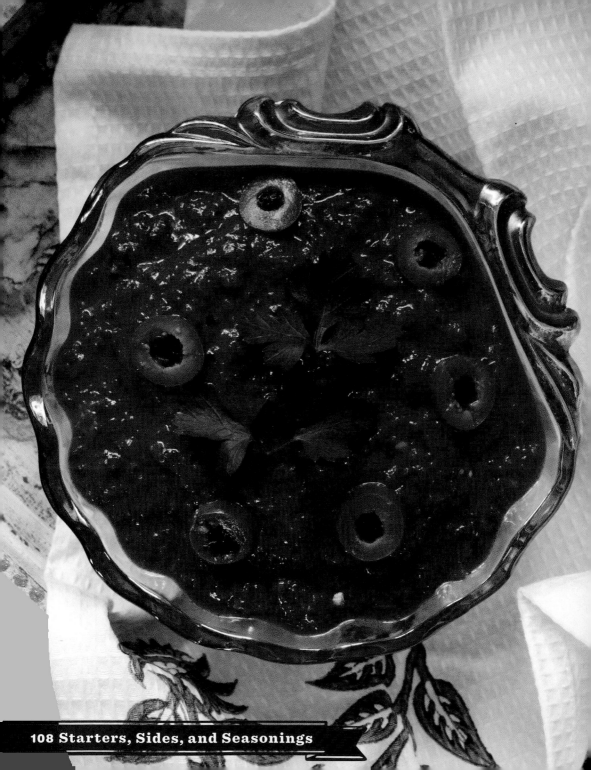

Roasted Bell Pepper Dip

YIELD: 4 SERVINGS • PREP TIME: 5 MINUTES • COOK TIME: 10 TO 20 MINUTES
NUTRITIONAL INFO: CALORIES: 68 • FAT: 8G • NET CARBS: 5G • PROTEIN: 2G

Fire-roasted peppers add depth to this rich and creamy dip.

1 Roast the bell peppers on the stove or over an open flame for about 10 minutes or until charred, making sure to rotate for even cooking. Alternatively, you can roast them in the oven for about 20 minutes at the highest temperature.

2 Cover peppers with foil and allow to cool. This will make it easier to remove the skins. When cool enough to handle, remove the skin and seeds from the peppers.

3 In food processor, blend the peppers with all the other ingredients until a smooth dip forms. Garnish with chopped olives and parsley, and serve.

INGREDIENTS

1 yellow bell pepper

1 red bell pepper

1 green bell pepper

2 tablespoons tahini

3 garlic cloves

1 tablespoon parsley

4 pitted olives

Salt, to taste

1 tablespoon olive oil

1 teaspoon paprika

Chili flakes, to taste

Chopped olives, for garnish

Parsley, for garnish

Smoky BBQ Sauce

This sauce is filled with intense spice and goes great when served on or alongside barbecued beef and pork dishes. The habanero pepper is optional in this recipe and should only be used by those who like their BBQ sauces hot!

INGREDIENTS

2 cups wood chips of choice

4 tablespoons butter

2 garlic cloves, finely chopped

1 medium white onion, finely chopped

4 tomatoes, finely chopped

¼ cup tomato paste

¼ cup white wine vinegar

¼ cup balsamic vinegar

2 tablespoons Dijon mustard

1 medium lime, juiced

2 tablespoons ginger, finely chopped

1 teaspoon smoked paprika

½ teaspoon ground cinnamon

2 dried chipotle peppers, finely chopped

1 habanero pepper, seeded and finely chopped (optional)

1 cup water

Salt and pepper, to taste

1 An hour before grilling, add the wood chips into a bowl of water and let soak.

2 Prepare your gas or charcoal grill to medium-high heat.

3 While waiting for the grill to heat up, place a small frying pan over medium heat and, when hot, add the butter, garlic, and onion and cook until the garlic has browned and the onion is translucent. Remove and set aside.

4 Transfer the cooked garlic and onion into a food processor, followed by the tomatoes and tomato paste. Puree into a thick paste, and then add the remaining ingredients to the food processor and blend thoroughly. Transfer the sauce into a medium saucepan and set alongside the grill.

5 When the grill is ready, about 400°F to 450°F with the coals lightly covered with ash, drain 1 cup of the wood chips and spread over the coals or pour in a smoker box. Place the medium saucepan on the grill and then bring the sauce to a boil with the grill covered, aligning the air vent away from the wood chips so that their smoke rolls around the sauce before escaping. Let the sauce cook for about 30 to 45 minutes, adding more wood chips every 20 minutes, until the sauce has reduced to about 2 cups.

6 Remove the sauce from the heat and serve warm. The sauce can be kept refrigerated for up to 2 weeks.

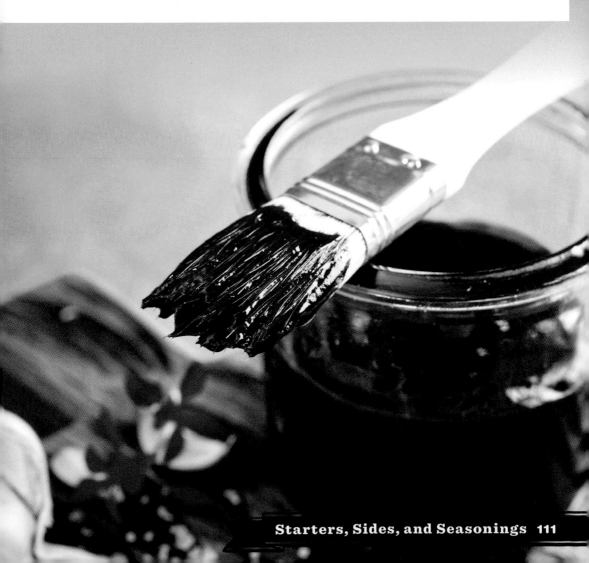

Barbecue Rub

YIELD: 4 TO 6 SERVINGS • PREP TIME: 2 MINUTES

NUTRITIONAL INFO: CALORIES: 9 • FAT: 0G • NET CARBS: 1G • PROTEIN: 0G

A simple rub can make all the difference when barbecuing something, whether it be half a zucchini or a steak. This one is particularly nice because it works with all diets.

INGREDIENTS

1 teaspoon cumin

1 teaspoon paprika

1 teaspoon garlic powder

1 teaspoon onion powder

1 teaspoon chili powder

1 teaspoon salt

¼ teaspoon ground black pepper

1 Mix ingredients together in a small bowl and apply generously to meats or vegetables, or store in an airtight container at room temperature for up to 1 month.

Garlic and Pepper Dry Rub

YIELD: 4 SERVINGS • PREP TIME: 2 MINUTES

NUTRITIONAL INFO: CALORIES: 11 • FAT: 0G • NET CARBS: 2G • PROTEIN: 0G

This rub is a little on the spicy side, so use sparingly unless you're a fan of heat.

INGREDIENTS

2 garlic cloves, minced

2 teaspoons fresh thyme, finely chopped

2 teaspoons salt

1½ teaspoons ground black pepper

1½ teaspoons ground white pepper

1 teaspoon ground red pepper

1 teaspoon sweet paprika

½ teaspoon onion powder

1 Mix ingredients together in a small bowl and apply generously to meats or vegetables, or store in an airtight container at room temperature for up to 1 month.

Tennessee Rub

YIELD: 4 SERVINGS • PREP TIME: 2 MINUTES
NUTRITIONAL INFO: CALORIES: 28 • FAT: 0G • NET CARBS: 2G • PROTEIN: 1G

This very strong rub is perfect when you are grilling up some beef or pork ribs. Knead the rub firmly into the meaty parts of the ribs to better impart its flavors.

INGREDIENTS

2 tablespoons ground black pepper

1 tablespoon smoked paprika

2 teaspoons yellow mustard seeds

2 teaspoons salt

1 teaspoon ground cumin

1 teaspoon dried oregano

1 teaspoon garlic powder

½ teaspoon cayenne pepper

1 Mix ingredients together in a small bowl and apply generously to meats or vegetables, or store in an airtight container at room temperature for up to 1 month.

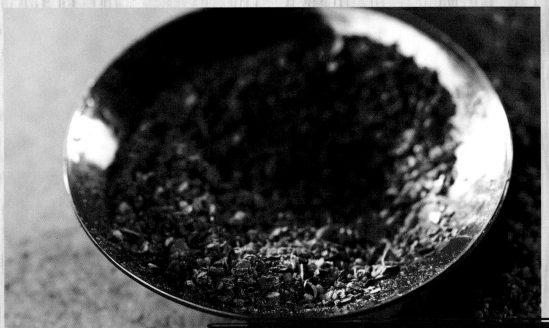

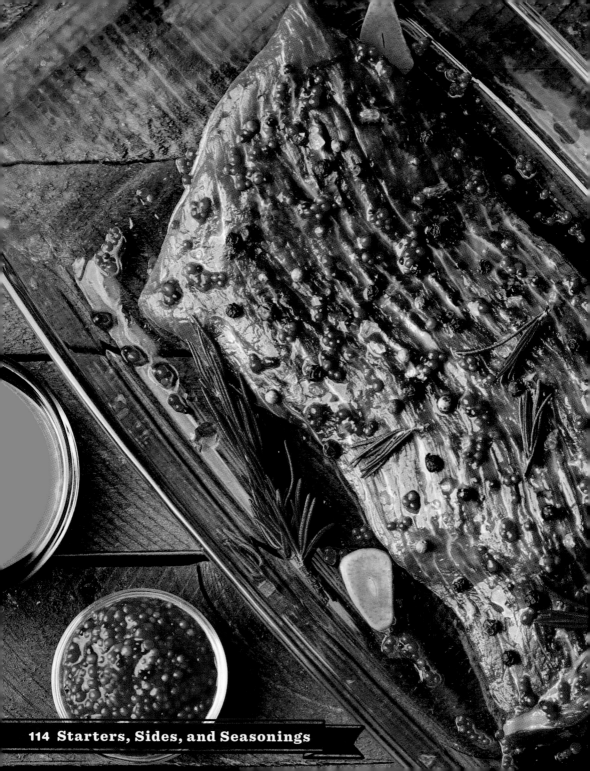

Balsamic and Dijon Marinade

YIELD: 4 SERVINGS • PREP TIME: 2 MINUTES
NUTRITIONAL INFO: CALORIES: 126 • FAT: 14G • NET CARBS: 1G • PROTEIN: 0G

The acidic and just a little sweet balsamic flavor pairs so well with vegetables—especially if they've had time to marinate prior to being grilled or tossed. Try this with zucchini, tomatoes, eggplants, or any salad.

1 Mix the ingredients in a small bowl and apply generously to meats or vegetables.

INGREDIENTS

4 tablespoons extra virgin olive oil

2 tablespoons balsamic vinegar

2 tablespoons lemon juice

1 tablespoon Dijon mustard

2 garlic cloves, minced

Salt and pepper, to taste

Lemon Marinade with Parsley and Red Bell Pepper

YIELD: 4 SERVINGS • PREP TIME: 4 HOURS 15 MINUTES
NUTRITIONAL INFO: CALORIES: 106 • FAT: 113G • NET CARBS: 10G • PROTEIN: 2G

Use this marinade for quick, last-minute meals, especially seafood dishes, as both the lemon and parsley flavors are mild when grilled.

INGREDIENTS

Juice of 2 medium lemons

2 garlic cloves, finely chopped

¼ cup fresh parsley, finely chopped

¼ cup fresh basil, finely chopped

1 tablespoon red bell pepper, finely chopped

1 tablespoon ground black pepper

2 teaspoons salt

½ cup extra virgin olive oil

1 In a medium bowl, combine all the ingredients and let rest for 15 minutes so the flavors can spread throughout the marinade.

2 To marinate, add meat or vegetable to the marinade and let rest for 4 hours, turning halfway through if not fully covered.

Olive Oil Infused with Rosemary

YIELD: 8 SERVINGS • PREP TIME: 1 TO 2 HOURS • COOK TIME: 5 MINUTES
NUTRITIONAL INFO: CALORIES: 242 • FAT: 28G • NET CARBS: 0G • PROTEIN: 0G

The soft flavors of rosemary always go well with a rib roast and its sides. It's extremely simple to infuse oil, and always worth it.

1 In a small saucepan, combine the rosemary, extra virgin olive oil, salt, and pepper, and place on the stovetop with the heat off. Set the heat to medium-low and let the oil heat, but do not let it reach a boil. Once hot, turn the heat off and let the rosemary infuse into the oil for 1 to 2 hours.

2 Strain the oil into a jar and keep at room temperature or in the refrigerator. Store for 2 or 4 months, respectively.

INGREDIENTS

6 large sprigs fresh rosemary

1 cup extra virgin olive oil

Salt and pepper, to taste

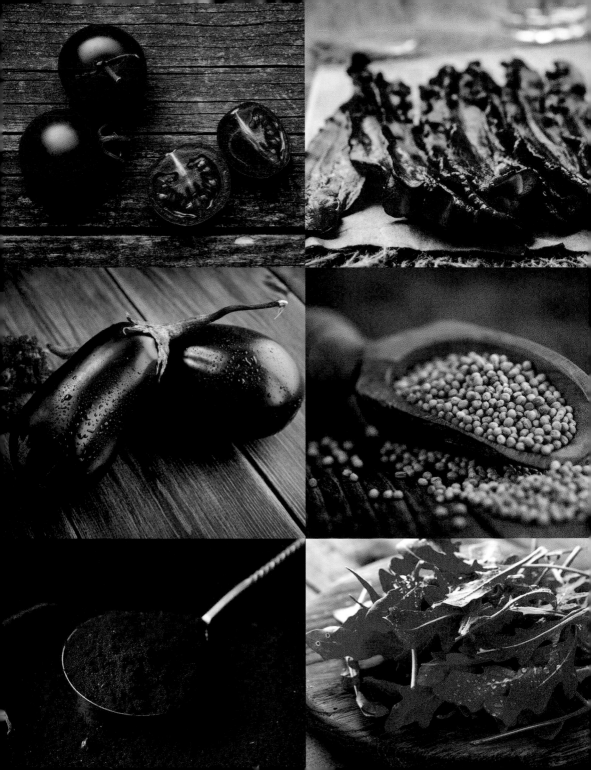

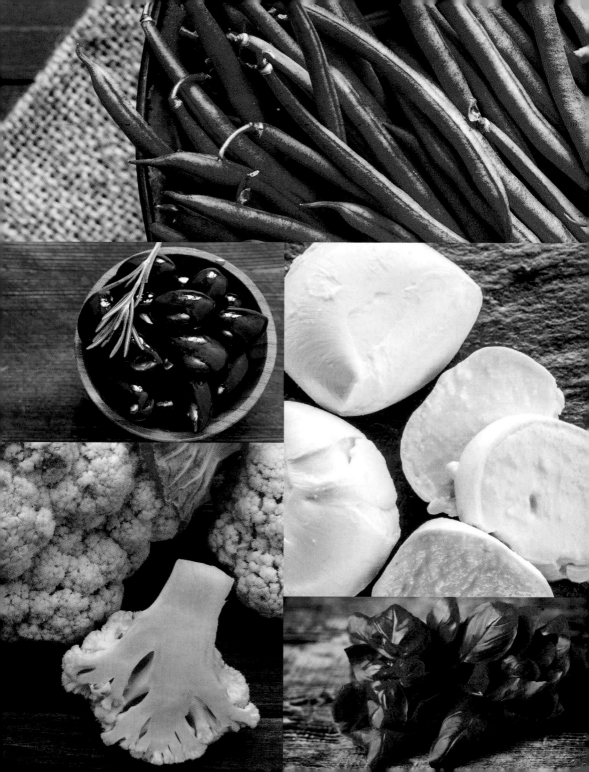

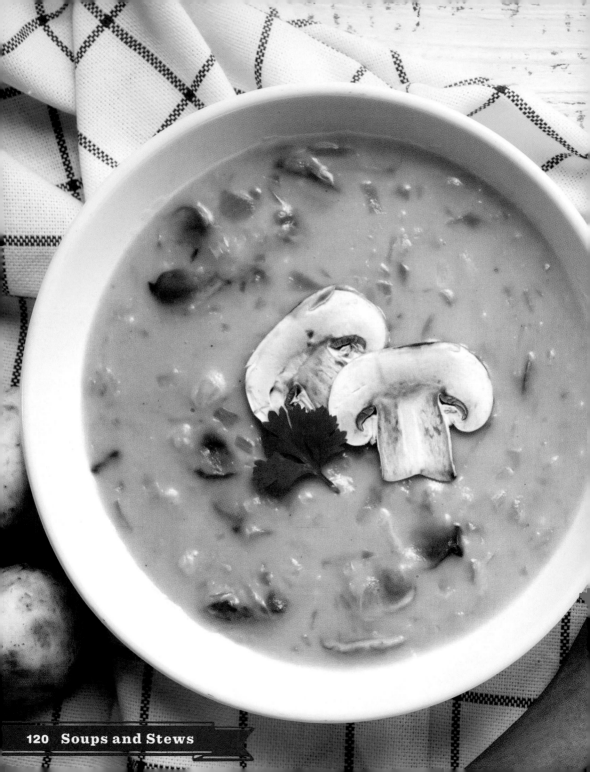

Soups and Stews

When eating keto you'll find you're doing a lot more cooking to avoid the hidden carbs in store-bought food and restaurant meals. This is where soups and stews step in. For starters, they're great comfort food—there's nothing quite like wolfing down a bowl of hot soup on a cold winter day. More importantly, they're easy to make.

For soups and stews, it's good to know how to make a great stock, because that forms the base of both. They are also a great way to get your vegetables in, something you can miss out on in keto because you're trying to up your fat and protein macros. Veggies are important because they give you nutrients and vitamins that you're not going to get just from meat and dairy. They're also your main source of carbohydrates on this diet, providing just enough to balance out your macros.

Stews are some of most flavorful dishes that can be created using the cheaper and tougher cuts of meat. The slow-cooking process allows the meat to break down and the flavor to really build up. Okay, so you can't mop it all up with bread, but some keto bread or Riced Cauliflower (page 81) will be the perfect accompaniment.

So throw a stew or soup on and let it fill your home with its lovely aromas while you go about doing your chores. Who said keto is hard?

Chicken Stock

YIELD: 6 QUARTS • PREP TIME: 10 MINUTES
COOK TIME: 5 TO 6 HOURS
NUTRITIONAL INFO: CALORIES: 18 • FAT: 2G • NET CARBS: 1G • PROTEIN: 2G

Be aware that stocks must cook slower to get the best flavor. Make sure to save the excess fat for an added boost in future recipes. Since this recipe makes a lot of stock, feel free to freeze some for later.

INGREDIENTS

10 lbs. chicken carcasses and/or stewing chicken pieces

½ cup vegetable oil

1 large yellow onion, unpeeled, cleaned root, cut into 1-inch pieces

1 celery stalk with leaves, cut into 1-inch pieces

10 quarts water

1 teaspoon salt

8 sprigs parsley

5 sprigs thyme

2 bay leaves

1 teaspoon peppercorns

1 Preheat oven to 350°F.

2 Lay the chicken carcasses and/or stewing pieces on a flat baking tray, place in oven, and cook for 30 to 45 minutes until golden brown. Remove and set aside.

3 Meanwhile, in a large stockpot, add the vegetable oil and warm over low heat. Add the vegetables and cook until any additional moisture has evaporated. This allows the flavor of the vegetables to become concentrated.

4 Add the water and the salt to the stockpot. Add the chicken carcasses and/or stewing pieces and the aromatics to the stockpot, raise heat to high, and bring to a boil.

5 Reduce heat so that the stock simmers and cook for a minimum of 2 hours. Skim fat and impurities from the top as the stock cooks. Cook for between 4 to 5 hours total.

6 When the stock is finished cooking, strain through a fine sieve or cheesecloth and place stock in refrigerator to chill.

7 Once cool, skim the fat layer from the top and save for future recipes. Use immediately, refrigerate, or freeze.

Fish Stock

YIELD: 10 CUPS • PREP TIME: 10 MINUTES • COOK TIME: 14 TO 23 HOURS
NUTRITIONAL INFO: CALORIES: 41 • FAT: 2G • NET CARBS: 0G • PROTEIN: 5G

Make a more delicate seafood stock using lobster bodies from which the claws and tails have been removed. For this recipe, use 3 to 4 lobster bodies, or the bodies of 2 lobsters and the shells from 2 to 4 pounds of raw shrimp.

1 Place the carcasses in the slow cooker. Cover with the water, vinegar, and clarified butter. Add the bay leaf and other aromatics.

2 Cover and cook on High for 4 to 5 hours until liquid is boiling. Remove the cover and scoop off and skim the impurities that have risen to the top.

3 Replace the cover and cook on Low for 10 to 18 hours— the longer the better.

4 Once cooking is complete, remove the solids with a slotted spoon. Transfer the stock to a large bowl and refrigerate. When the fat is congealed on top, remove it and set aside, and transfer the stock to several smaller containers with tight-fitting lids. Stock can be stored in the refrigerator for several days or frozen.

INGREDIENTS

2 or 3 whole carcasses from non-oily fish (such as snapper, rockfish, sole, or cod)

3 quarts cold water

¼ cup vinegar

2 tablespoons clarified butter

1 bay leaf

3 sprigs thyme

3 sprigs parsley

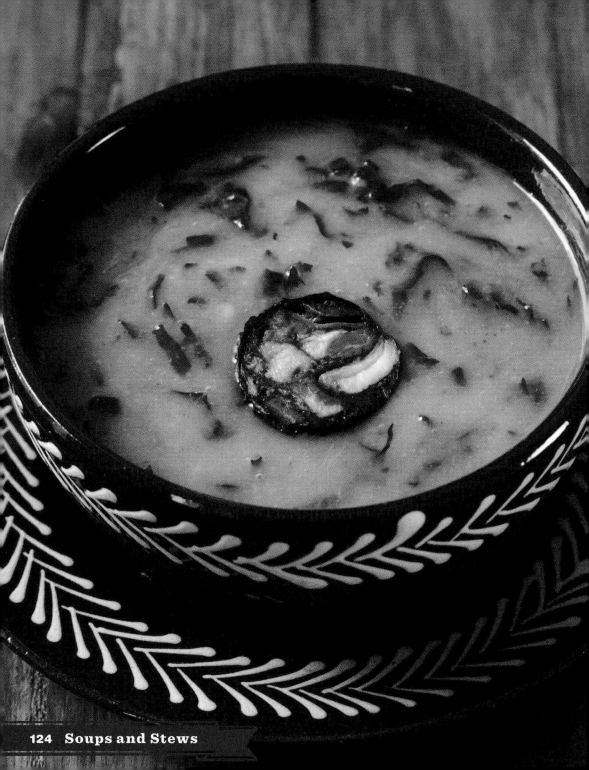

Homemade Sausage and Kale Soup

YIELD: 6 SERVINGS • PREP TIME: 15 MINUTES • COOK TIME: 35 MINUTES
NUTRITIONAL INFO: CALORIES: 281 • FAT: 21G • NET CARBS: 8G • PROTEIN: 18G

Keto-friendly sausage can be hard to come by. However, if you go to your local farmers market or butcher, you should be able to find a sausage that works for your diet. It will be worth it, especially in this traditional Portuguese soup.

1 Place a large Dutch oven on your gas or charcoal grill and prepare to medium heat. Leave the grill covered while heating, as it will add a faint smoky flavor to the pot.

2 When the grill is ready, at about 400°F with the coals lightly covered with ash, add the oil into the Dutch oven, followed by the onion, garlic, and sausage pieces. Cook until the onion and sausage have browned, about 7 minutes. Remove the sausage from the pan and set aside.

3 Next, stir in the pepper flakes, chicken stock, and water and bring to a boil. Cook, uncovered, for about 20 minutes. Add in the kale and boil for about 5 more minutes until tender. Stir in the sausage and cook for about 2 more minutes.

4 Remove the Dutch oven from the grill and season with salt and pepper. Serve hot.

INGREDIENTS

2 tablespoons olive oil

½ onion, finely chopped

1 garlic clove, finely chopped

¾ lb. pork sausage, cut into ½-inch pieces

¼ teaspoon red pepper flakes

3 cups chicken stock

2 cups water

1 lb. fresh kale, stemmed and chopped

Salt and pepper, to taste

Red Wine Beef Stew

YIELD: 8 SERVINGS • PREP TIME: 10 MINUTES • COOK TIME: 6 TO 10 HOURS
NUTRITIONAL INFO: CALORIES: 398 • FAT: 17G • NET CARBS: 12G • PROTEIN: 50G

Since this dish has more protein than fat, it might make sense to add a tablespoon of butter per portion to hit your daily macros. At 12 net carbs, this dish is a bit higher than most keto dishes, but if you make the stew without the wine it will result in a much lower carb count.

INGREDIENTS

4 tablespoons olive oil

2 cloves garlic, minced

4 lbs. chuck roast, cut into ½-inch pieces

1 onion, sliced thin

½ cup fresh mushrooms, sliced

1 teaspoon dried rosemary

Salt and pepper, to taste

1 cup dry red wine

2 cups water

1 Heat the oil in a skillet and add the garlic. Cook the beef in the oil until lightly browned on all sides. Transfer to the slow cooker.

2 Add the onion to the skillet and cook, stirring, until onions are translucent, about 3 minutes. Add the mushrooms and stir, cooking for another minute or so. Remove from heat and add the rosemary. Season the mixture with salt and pepper and add to the slow cooker.

3 Pour the wine and water over everything in the slow cooker. Cover and cook on Low for 8 to 10 hours or on High for 6 to 7 hours.

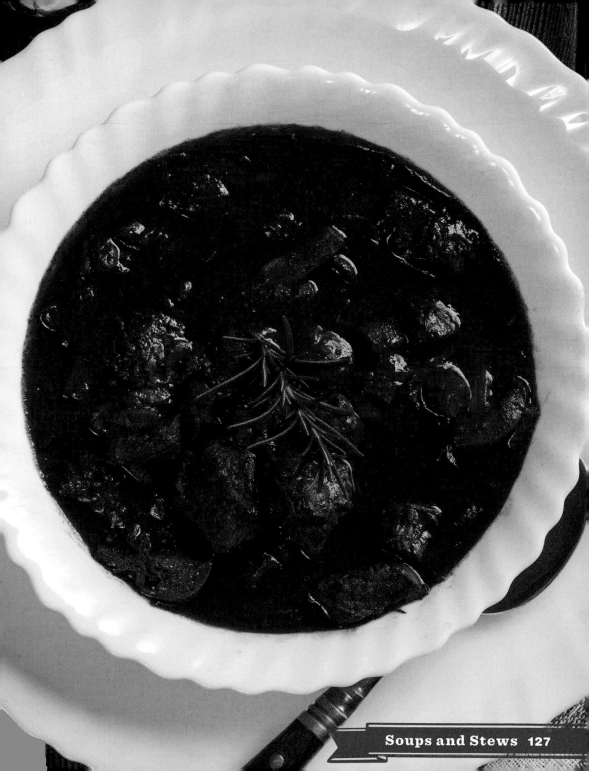

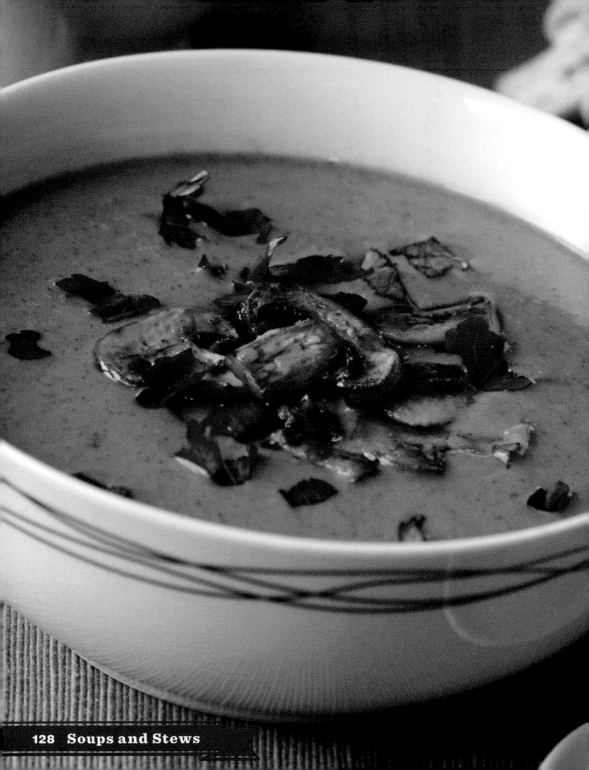

Bacon Mushroom Soup

YIELD: 8 SERVINGS • PREP TIME: 5 MINUTES • COOK TIME: 3 TO 6 HOURS
NUTRITIONAL INFO: CALORIES: 224 • FAT: 16G • NET CARBS: 6G • PROTEIN: 12G

The recipe calls for thick-cut bacon so that you get larger pieces, but you can use any kind of bacon. If you're looking for an added kick, try using bacon that has been smoked.

1 In a skillet over medium heat, cook the bacon pieces, stirring frequently, until the bacon is crisp. Remove the meat from the pan, placing it on a paper towel over a plate to absorb some of the fat, then place back into the pan.

2 Add the onion to the skillet and cook while stirring until the onion starts to wilt, about 2 minutes. Add the sage and cayenne and stir. Remove from heat.

3 Put the sliced fresh mushrooms in the slow cooker. Add the bacon-and-onion mixture. Add the dried porcini mushrooms and top with the broth. Stir to combine. Cover and cook on Low for 5 to 6 hours or on High for about 3 hours.

4 Stir in the heavy cream and season with salt and pepper to taste.

INGREDIENTS

6 strips thick-cut bacon, diced

½ cup chopped yellow onion

½ teaspoon dried sage

¼ teaspoon cayenne pepper

½ lb. fresh shiitake mushrooms, stems removed, sliced

½ lb. fresh cremini mushrooms, stems removed, sliced

1 lb. fresh baby portobello mushrooms, stems removed, sliced

1 oz. dried porcini mushrooms

3½ cups chicken broth

1 cup heavy cream

Salt and pepper, to taste

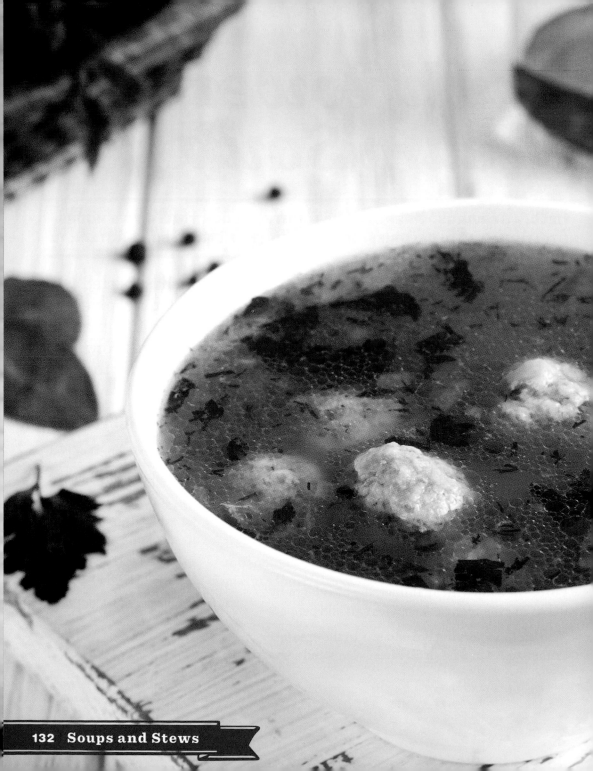

Ground Turkey and Broccoli Stew

YIELD: 8 SERVINGS • PREP TIME: 10 MINUTES
COOK TIME: 2 HOURS 10 MINUTES TO 6 HOURS 10 MINUTES
NUTRITIONAL INFO: CALORIES: 293 • FAT: 14G • NET CARBS: 5G • PROTEIN: 22G

Brown and cook these turkey meatballs in the skillet before putting them in the slow cooker and put the vegetables and broth around them. For more richness and fat, add in some heavy cream.

1 In a large skillet over medium-high heat, cook the onion and garlic in the oil for 3 to 4 minutes. Sprinkle the cumin over the mixture and continue stirring and cooking another minute or so.

2 Add ground turkey and cook until meat is browned, about 5 minutes.

3 Put mixture into the slow cooker. Top with the frozen broccoli and the stock. Cover and cook on Low for 5 to 6 hours or on High for 2 to 3 hours. Season with salt and pepper to taste.

INGREDIENTS

½ onion, chopped

2 garlic cloves, minced

2 tablespoons olive oil

1 teaspoon ground cumin

1 lb. ground turkey

16 oz. package frozen broccoli

3 cups chicken or vegetable stock

Salt and pepper, to taste

Bouillabaisse

YIELD: 8 SERVINGS • PREP TIME: 15 MINUTES
COOK TIME: 3 HOURS 45 MINUTES TO 6 HOURS
NUTRITIONAL INFO: CALORIES: 170 • FAT: 6G • NET CARBS: 4G • PROTEIN: 26G

This classic French fish "boil" is said to have originated in the seaside town of Marseilles in the south of France. The word itself has a fanciful attribution—*bouille-besse*, or the Abbess' Boil—in reference to a particular Abbess in a convent there, as well as the more practical *bouillon abaissé*, meaning, "to reduce by evaporation." To increase the fat content of this dish, add in a tablespoon of butter to each serving. Alternatively, heavy cream can be added as well, depending on your preference.

INGREDIENTS

½ onion, chopped

2 garlic cloves, minced

1 celery stalk, fronds removed, stalk finely chopped

1 red bell pepper, seeded and chopped

1 cup fish stock (or clam juice)

½ cup water

2 tablespoons extra virgin olive oil

1 tablespoon lemon zest

1 tablespoon fresh basil, chopped

1 tablespoon fresh parsley, chopped

1 teaspoon fresh oregano

1 teaspoon fresh thyme

1 bay leaf

1 lb. firm white fish, cut into 1-inch pieces

¾ lb. shelled, cleaned shrimp, tails removed if preferred

6.5 oz. can chopped clams and juice

8 oz. cleaned, fresh crabmeat

Salt, to taste

¼ cup fresh parsley, chopped, for garnish

1 In a large bowl, combine onion, garlic, celery, red pepper, fish stock, water, olive oil, lemon zest, herbs, and bay leaf. Mix well. Put into slow cooker.

2 Cover and cook on Low for 4 to 5 hours or on High for 2 to 3 hours until base is hot and flavors are combined.

3 Stir in fish, shrimp, clams, and crab and cook for an additional 45 minutes to 1 hour or until fish is done (if cooking on High, reduce heat to Low). Remove bay leaf before serving. Season with salt to taste and garnish with parsley.

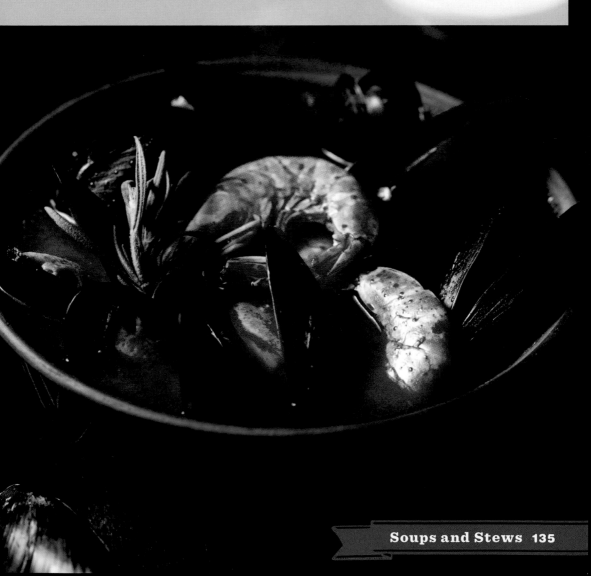

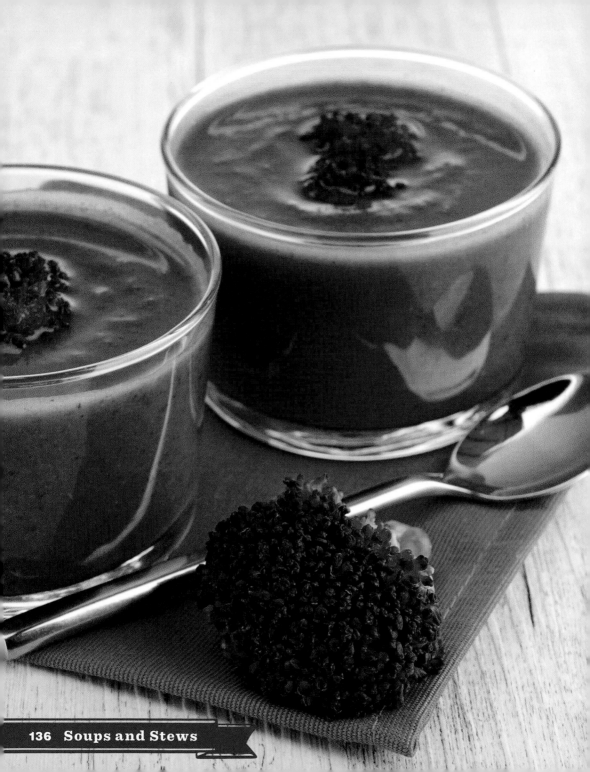

Curry Soup with Broccoli

YIELD: 4 SERVINGS • PREP TIME: 5 MINUTES • COOK TIME: 4 TO 6 HOURS
NUTRITIONAL INFO: CALORIES: 290 • FAT: 23G • NET CARBS: 7G • PROTEIN: 8G

The addition of the baking soda will help maintain the bright green color of the broccoli through the long cooking process. The heavy cream can be substituted with coconut cream, if you prefer.

1 In a skillet over medium heat, cook the onion in the butter until translucent, 2 to 3 minutes. Remove from heat and stir in the curry powder.

2 Transfer the onion mixture to the slow cooker. Add the broccoli. Stir the baking soda into the chicken broth until dissolved and pour over broccoli. Cover and cook on Low for 6 hours or on High for 4 hours.

3 Add in the heavy cream, then use a hand-held blender to puree the soup, or process it in batches in a blender. Season with salt and pepper and serve.

INGREDIENTS

¼ onion, chopped

4 tablespoons unsalted butter

1 teaspoon curry powder

1 lb. broccoli florets, tough stems removed

1 teaspoon baking soda

3 cups chicken broth

½ cup heavy cream

Salt and pepper, to taste

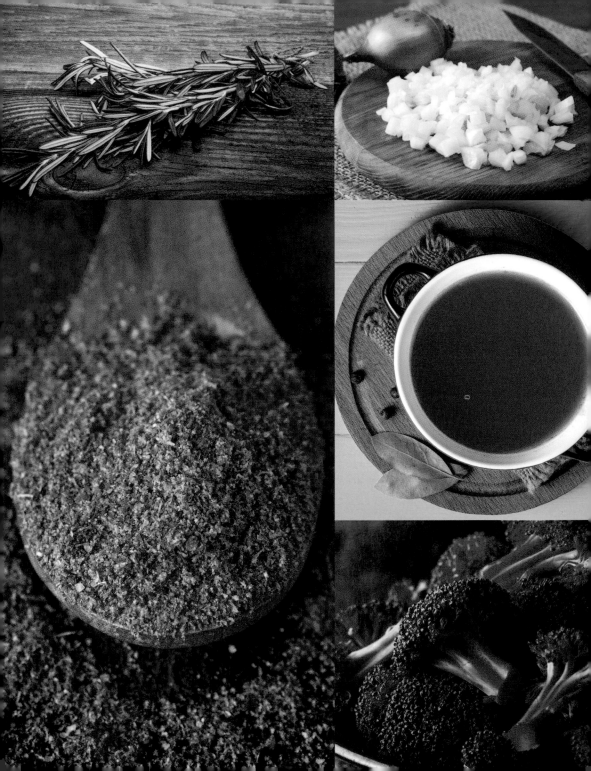

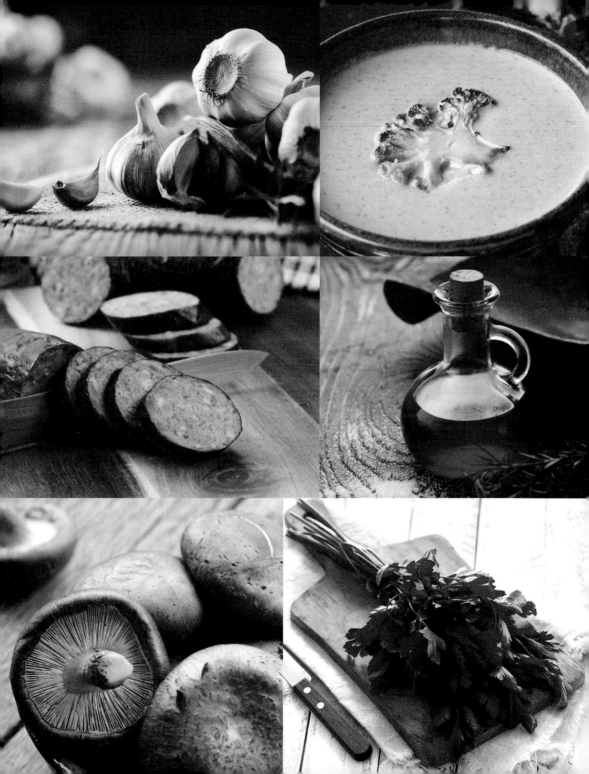

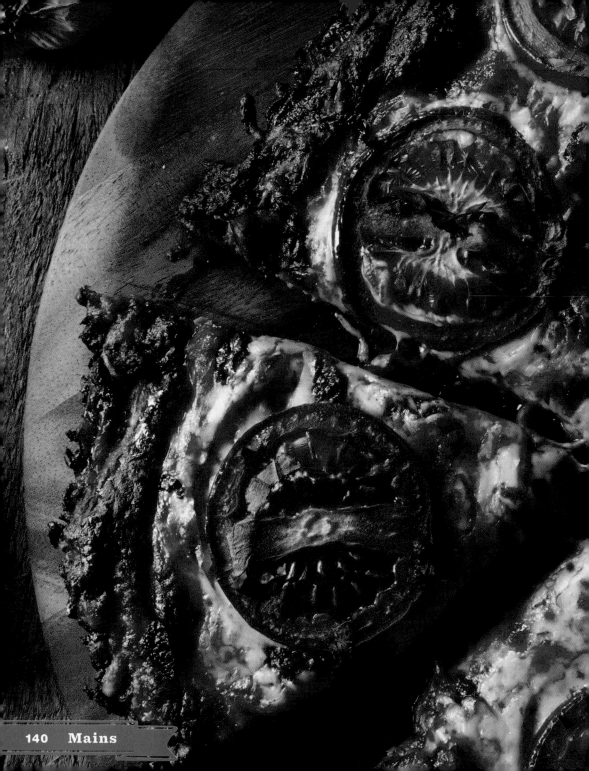

Mains

On the keto diet, people seem to think that mains are just big hunks of meat drowned in butter and oil—but they're much more than that. There's no reason your main course can't be an incredible dish, well balanced and full of flavor, and it's surprising how many "regular" foods lend themselves to keto—think Pork Vindaloo (page 173), Chicken Parmigiana (page 194), or Slow Cooker Turkey Meatballs and Zucchini (page 209). Hankering after an unhealthy pizza? Sub in eggplant slices or portobello mushrooms for a delicious veggie "pizza," or go a step further and make Cauliflower Pizza Dough (page 248).

No time to cook an elaborate meal on a weekday? Seafood mains are quick to cook and chock-full of Omega-3 fats and healthy protein and will come together in minutes. Eating alone? A single serving of the Grilled Chicken Breast with Sesame Seeds and Ginger (page 196) is just the ticket. For those relaxing weekends when you're putting together a week's worth of meals, there are great slow cooker recipes that you can throw together overnight and wake up to a delicious dish the next day. And if you'd really just like a big hunk of meat, the Argentinian Chimichurri Porterhouse Steak (page 142) or Prime Rib Roast (page 158) are both easy and achievable.

Argentinian Chimichurri Porterhouse Steak

YIELD: 4 SERVINGS • PREP TIME: 1 HOUR 25 MINUTES COOK TIME: 20 MINUTES
NUTRITIONAL INFO (FOR THE STEAK): CALORIES: 479 • FAT: 39G • NET CARBS: 0G •
PROTEIN: 30G
NUTRITIONAL INFO (FOR THE SAUCE): CALORIES: 396 • FAT: 42G • NET CARBS: 4G •
PROTEIN: 1G

The Argentinian Chimichurri sauce goes well with any steak. It can be used as a marinade, though this is sometimes a little risky because of the light kick from the Fresno chili. For those who would like even more heat in the sauce, substitute a habanero in place of the Fresno chili.

INGREDIENTS

For the Steak

2 porterhouse steaks, about 1½ inches thick (21 oz. weight total)

4 tablespoons extra virgin olive oil

Salt and pepper, to taste

For the Argentinian Chimichurri

½ cup red wine vinegar

4 garlic cloves, minced

1 shallot, minced

½ scallion, minced

1 Fresno chili, finely chopped

1 tablespoon fresh lemon juice

1 teaspoon salt

½ cup flat-leaf parsley, minced

½ cup cilantro, minced

2 tablespoons oregano, minced

¾ cup extra virgin olive oil

1 Rub both sides of the steaks with oil and let rest at room temperature for about 1 hour.

2 A half hour before cooking, prepare your gas or charcoal grill to medium-high heat.

3 While you wait, to make the sauce, combine the vinegar, garlic, shallot, scallion, Fresno chili, lemon juice, and salt in a medium bowl and let rest for 15 minutes. Next, add the parsley, cilantro, and oregano, then gradually whisk in the oil. Set aside.

4 When the grill is ready, at about 400°F to 450°F with the coals lightly covered with ash, season one side of the steaks with salt and pepper, as well as a very light brush of the sauce along the bone.

5 Place the seasoned sides of the steaks on the grill and cook for about 5 to 6 minutes, seasoning the tops of the steaks while waiting. Again, lightly trace the bone with the sauce. Once the steaks are charred, flip and cook for 4 to 5 more minutes for medium-rare, and 6 to 7 for medium. The steaks should feel slightly firm if poked in the center.

6 Remove the steaks from the grill and transfer to a large cutting board. Let stand for 10 minutes, allowing the steaks to properly store their juices and flavor. Serve warm with the sauce on the side.

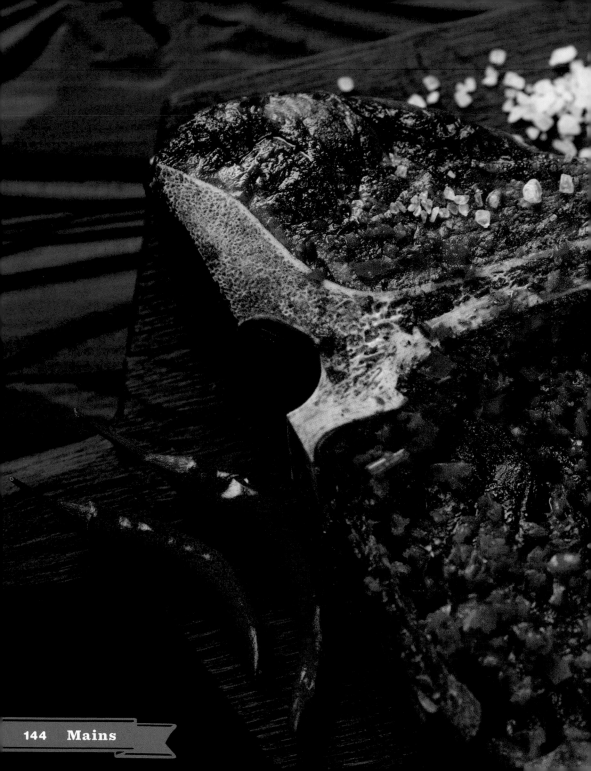

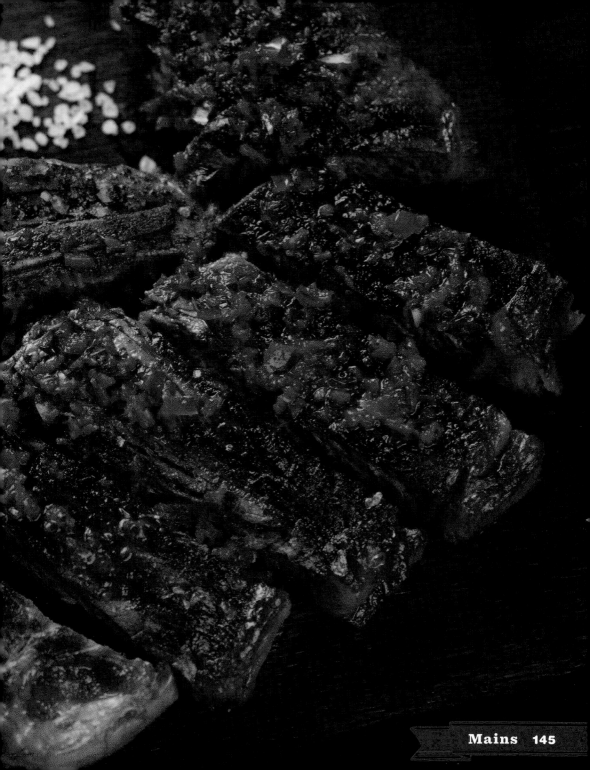

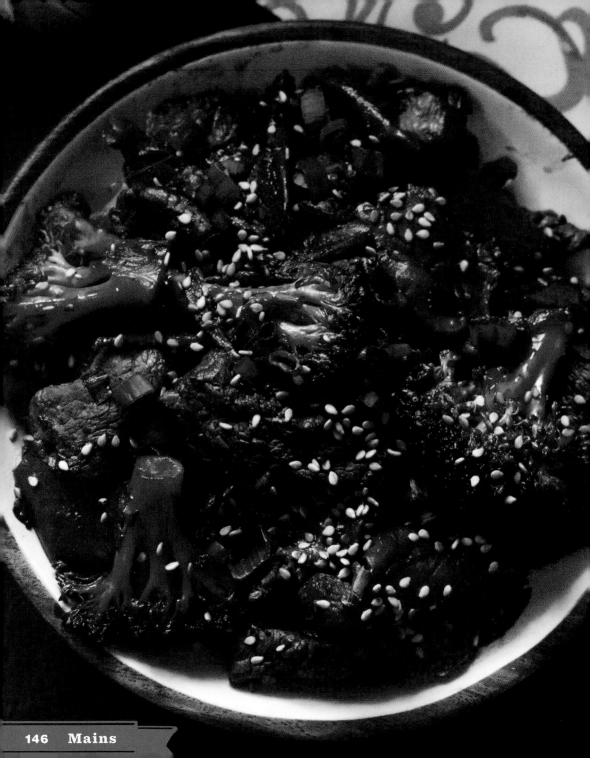

Beef and Broccoli Stir Fry

YIELD: 2 SERVINGS • PREP TIME: 5 MINUTES • COOK TIME: 10 MINUTES
NUTRITIONAL INFO: CALORIES: 466 • FAT: 32G • NET CARBS: 5G • PROTEIN: 37G

The oyster mushrooms provide a noodly toothiness to this Asian-style stir fry.

1 Heat the oil and butter in a wok and stir fry the spring onion whites, ginger, and garlic. Add in the mushrooms and sauté until they start to caramelize.

2 Add in the beef and continue frying; season with salt, pepper, and five-spice powder.

3 Microwave the broccoli for 2 minutes and add it to the wok, then add the vinegar, soy sauce, and spring onion greens. Season to taste, stir fry for another minute, and garnish with sesame seeds before serving.

INGREDIENTS

1 tablespoon olive oil

1 tablespoon unsalted butter

1 spring onion, chopped (white and green sections separated)

1 teaspoon ginger

1 teaspoon garlic, chopped

1¼ cups oyster mushrooms

8 oz. beef tenderloin, cut into strips

Salt and pepper, to taste

Five-spice powder, to taste

½ cup broccoli florets

1 tablespoon vinegar

1 tablespoon soy sauce

Sesame seeds, for garnish

Beef Rib Crown Roast

YIELD: 12 SERVINGS • PREP TIME: 1 TO 1½ HOURS
COOK TIME: ABOUT 2 TO 3 HOURS
NUTRITIONAL INFO: CALORIES: 966 • FAT: 83G • NET CARBS: 8G • PROTEIN: 87G

It can be difficult to get the beef ribs to form a crown roast, so make sure to use plenty of string.

INGREDIENTS

10-rib beef rib roast (about 10 lbs.)

3 tablespoons salt

3 tablespoons black pepper

1 cup extra virgin olive oil

8 garlic cloves, minced

⅓ cup fresh thyme, coarsely chopped

⅓ cup fresh rosemary, coarsely chopped

4 tablespoons fresh sage, finely chopped

1 Remove the rib roast from the refrigerator and place it on cooling racks over a large carving board, bone-side down. To begin, cut the meat that covers the bones. To do so, go about 2 inches down the ribs and using a sharp carving knife, cut through the meat until you reach the bone. Make a sharp cut and then cut up the bone so that the top of the meat can be peeled off. This process is known as "Frenching" in the culinary world.

2 Stand the rib roast up and, starting with the left bone, cut down 1 to 2 inches along the bone, across to the next bone, and then back up so that you get a rectangular chunk of the meat to come apart from the space between the ribs. Do this to all the ribs, and then gently cut away the meat so that the ribs are left to stand openly and on their own. Using a paring knife, gently scrape away any bits of meat that still cling to the ribs.

3 Bring the meat together into a circle and cut about ½ to 1 inch into the meat side of the rib roast between each bone. Make your cuts even and leveled. Stand the rib roast and, pushing back the ends of the roast, form it into a tight crown. Note that because it's fairly difficult to crown a roast of beef, you may need to cut deeper than 1 inch between the ribs for more flexibility. Using butcher's twine, tie the crown tightly so that it will remain in that position while roasting—you'll need to tie the roast around the bones themselves, and also around the equator of the roast. Set aside.

4 Mix the salt and pepper in a small bowl. Using your hands, massage the mixture into the rib roast.

5 In a small bowl, whisk together the remaining ingredients. Using your hands, massage the paste into the rib roast. Let stand at room temperature for 30 minutes to 1 hour.

6 Preheat the oven to 450°F. Place the standing rib roast in a large roasting pan. Cover the crown with aluminum foil so that it keeps the heat central. Roast at 450°F for 15 minutes so that the rib roast receives a nice initial searing.

7 Lower the heat to 325°F and cook for another 2 to 3 hours, until the internal temperature of the meat reads 125°F for medium-rare. Baste the rib roast with its own juices every 30 minutes or so.

8 Remove the crown roast from the oven and place on a large serving platter. Let stand for 10 minutes before carving.

Easy Prime Rib

YIELD: 4 TO 8 SERVINGS • PREP TIME: 2 HOURS 10 MINUTES • COOK TIME: 5 HOURS

NUTRITIONAL INFO: CALORIES: 686 • FAT: 47G • NET CARBS: 5G • PROTEIN: 53G

With the slow cooker, a low temperature cooks the meat over a longer period of time, requiring little to no effort on your part. It's not entirely necessary to baste the roast every 30 minutes. Instead, just make sure that the roast is at least half submerged in the liquid and that you cook it on the low setting. Other than that, let the slow cooker do all the work for you.

INGREDIENTS

3- or 4-rib beef rib roast (approx. 4 lbs.)

2 tablespoons salt

2 tablespoons black pepper

4 garlic cloves, minced

1 teaspoon extra virgin olive oil

4 sprigs fresh rosemary

4 sprigs fresh thyme

¼ cup dry red wine

1 cup chicken stock

1 bay leaf

1 Remove the rib roast from the refrigerator 1 hour before cooking. Using your hands, thoroughly apply the salt and pepper to the rib roast.

2 Next, in a small bowl, mix together the minced garlic and oil, and then apply to the roast. Let the roast stand at room temperature for about 1 hour.

3 Add the rosemary, thyme, red wine, chicken stock, and bay leaf to a slow cooker. Add the rib roast, fat side up, to the slow cooker. Turn the slow cooker to Low and let cook for about 5 hours until, when tested with an instant-read thermometer, the internal temperature reads 130°F for medium-rare. Note that the liquid will not completely cover the rib roast, so baste it or flip the meat halfway through the cooking time.

4 Remove the rib roast from the slow cooker and place on a large carving board. Let rest for 15 minutes before carving. As far as the leftover liquid goes, you can use this as the base of a sauce or gravy.

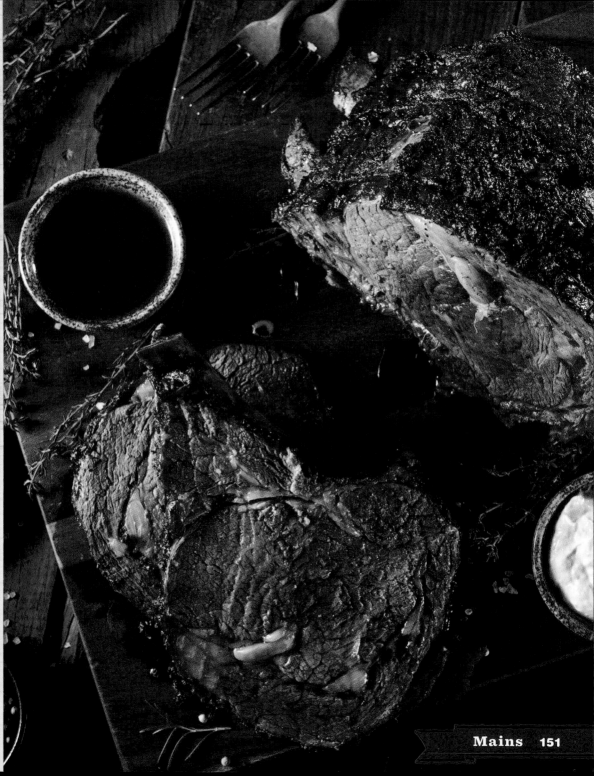

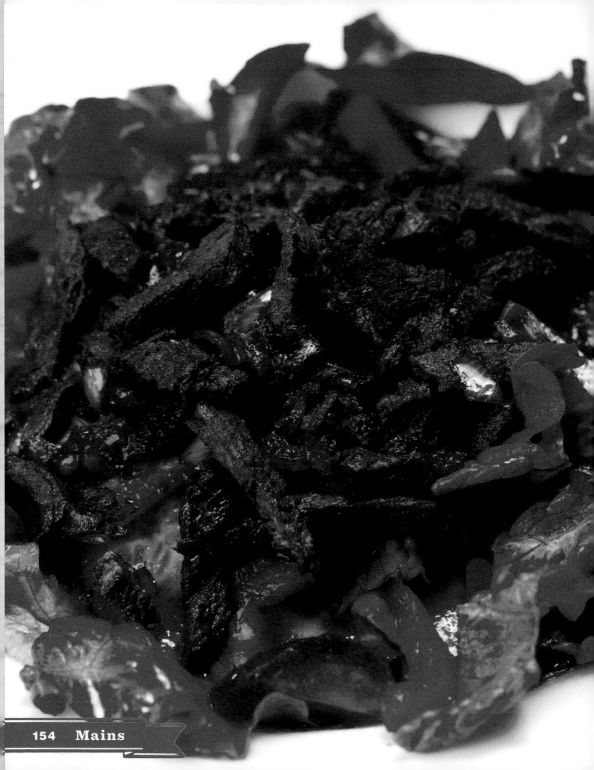

Lettuce-Wrapped Peppers and Beef

YIELD: 10 SERVINGS • PREP TIME: 5 MINUTES • COOK TIME: 5 TO 8 HOURS
NUTRITIONAL INFO: CALORIES: 261 • FAT: 16G • NET CARBS: 5G • PROTEIN: 22G

If you want to wrap the peppers and beef in something besides lettuce leaves, consider low-carb tortillas. For extra flavor, brush both sides with some oil and toast them on the grill for a minute or so a side. Macros do not include the lettuce or grated cheese on top, so make sure to log those per the quantity you use.

1 Heat the oil in a large skillet or saucepan. Add the onion and peppers and cook until just softening, about 5 minutes. Stir in the jalapeños and ancho chili powder.

2 Transfer pepper mixture to the slow cooker. Top with the slices of steak and pour the pureed tomatoes over everything. Cover and cook on Low for 6 to 8 hours, or on High for 5 to 6 hours until the steak is tender.

3 To serve, put the steak and pepper mixture in a bowl with a lid, and serve alongside a platter of prepared lettuce leaves. Fill the leaves as necessary so they don't get soggy and tear. Sprinkle grated cheese on top and serve.

INGREDIENTS

¼ cup extra virgin olive oil

1 small onion, chopped

1 each of medium-sized yellow, red, and green bell peppers, cored, seeded, and sliced

2 jalapeño peppers, diced

1 teaspoon ancho chili powder

2 to 3 lbs. sirloin beef, cut into thin strips

7 tomatoes, pureed

1 head crisp lettuce, like romaine or endive, cut or broken into 3-inch sections

Grated cheddar or pepper jack cheese, for garnish

Olive Tapenade Skirt Steak

YIELD: 4 SERVINGS • PREP TIME: 1 HOUR 10 MINUTES • COOK TIME: 10 MINUTES
NUTRITIONAL INFO: CALORIES: 1000 • FAT: 66G • NET CARBS: 5G • PROTEIN: 22G

The skirt steak is often referred to as the chewiest piece of meat. Because of how thin it is, it is very easy to overcook, which then increases the chewiness. As such, grill these steaks over direct heat and make sure not to cook past medium.

INGREDIENTS

For the Steak

2 skirt steaks (1 lb. each)

2 tablespoons extra virgin olive oil

Salt and pepper, to taste

For the Olive Tapenade

1 cup Niçoise olives, pitted and chopped

½ cup extra virgin olive oil

½ small shallot, minced

1 garlic clove, minced

1 sprig of rosemary, leaves removed and minced

1 anchovy fillet (optional)

1 tablespoon basil, finely chopped

1 tablespoon flat-leaf parsley, finely chopped

1 tablespoon capers, minced

1 tablespoon thyme

1 teaspoon red pepper flakes

1 Rub both sides of the steaks with oil and let rest at room temperature for about 1 hour.

2 While waiting, combine the tapenade ingredients in a medium bowl and mix thoroughly. Set aside.

3 A half hour before cooking, prepare your gas or charcoal grill to extremely high heat.

4 When the grill is ready, about 500°F to 600°F with the coals lightly covered with ash, season the steaks with salt and pepper. Place the steaks on the grill and spoon the tapenade onto the top of each steak. Cook for about 3 minutes and then flip. Again, add the tapenade and cook for about 2 to 3 minutes for medium-rare, and 3 to 4 for medium. The steaks should be very charred and slightly firm if poked in the center. If an instant-read thermometer is inserted into the thickest section of the meat it should read around 125°F.

5 Remove the steaks from the grill and transfer to a large cutting board. Let stand for 5 to 10 minutes. Slice the steaks diagonally into long, thin slices and arrange the remaining tapenade on the side. Serve warm.

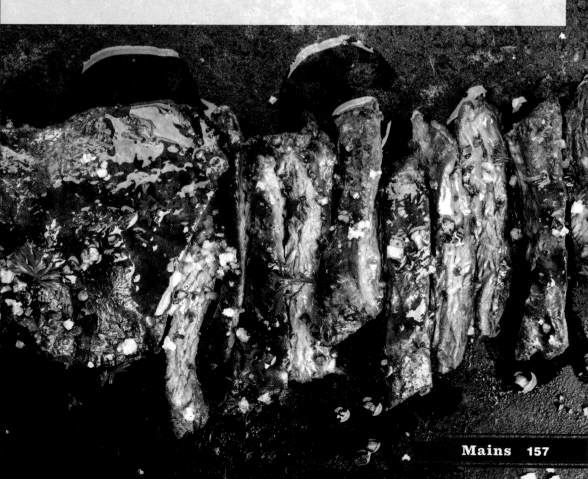

Prime Rib Roast

YIELD: 8 SERVINGS • PREP TIME: 1 HOUR 20 MINUTES
COOK TIME: 2 TO 3 HOURS
NUTRITIONAL INFO: CALORIES: 736 • FAT: 64G • NET CARBS: 0G • PROTEIN: 77G

If you really want to take it easy, throw the roast into a slow cooker—you don't even have the baste the meat. Just cover your roast, set your slow cooker to low, and relax.

INGREDIENTS

3 tablespoons salt

3 tablespoons ground black pepper

6-rib beef rib roast (approx. 6 lbs.)

¼ cup extra virgin olive oil

1 In a small bowl, combine the salt and pepper and mix thoroughly. Using your hands, pat the mixture firmly onto the rib roast and then brush with oil. Let stand at room temperature for 1 hour before cooking.

2 Set a large plancha skillet across two burners on the stovetop and set to high heat. You can also use a cast-iron skillet large enough to fit the rib roast. Place the rib roast fatty side down on the plancha skillet and sear for 15 minutes, until a crust forms. Once crusted, remove from the skillet and place on cooling racks set over a large carving board. Let rest for 15 minutes.

3 Preheat the oven to 325°F. Place the rib roast fat side down on a rack in a roasting pan and transfer to the oven. Roast for 2 to 3 hours, basting every 30 minutes or so with its own juices, until its internal temperature reads 125°F for medium-rare.

4 Remove the rib roast from the oven and let rest for 10 minutes before carving, allowing it to properly store its juices and flavor.

Rosemary and Thyme Flank Steak

YIELD: 2 SERVINGS • PREP TIME: 1 HOUR 10 MINUTES • COOK TIME: 15 MINUTES
NUTRITIONAL INFO: CALORIES: 584 • FAT: 44G • NET CARBS: 0G • PROTEIN: 48G

Due to the flank's toughness, it is essential to slice this steak into very thin strips.

1 Rub the steak with a mixture of the olive oil, rosemary, and thyme. Let rest at room temperature for 1 hour.

2 A half hour before cooking, prepare your gas or charcoal grill to medium-high heat.

3 When the grill is ready, about 400°F to 450°F with the coals lightly covered with ash, season one side of the steak with salt and pepper. Place the seasoned side of the steak on the grill and cook for about 4 to 5 minutes, seasoning the uncooked side of the steak while waiting. When the steak seems charred, gently flip and cook for 4 to 5 more minutes for medium-rare and 6 more minutes for medium. The steak should feel slightly firm if poked in the center.

4 Remove the steak from the grill and transfer to a large cutting board. Let stand for 6 to 8 minutes. Slice the steak diagonally into long, thin slices. Serve warm topped with the butter.

INGREDIENTS

1 flank steak (approx. 1 to 1½ lbs.)

2 tablespoons extra virgin olive oil

2 sprigs rosemary, leaves removed

2 sprigs thyme, leaves removed

Salt and pepper, to taste

2 tablespoons butter

Rib Eye with Chipotle Rub

YIELD: 2 TO 3 SERVINGS • PREP TIME: 1 HOUR 10 MINUTES
COOK TIME: 20 MINUTES
NUTRITIONAL INFO: CALORIES: 909 • FAT: 69G • NET CARBS: 8G • PROTEIN: 60G

To decrease the carbs, replace the chipotles with some cayenne pepper. For additional fat, top the finished steak with butter.

INGREDIENTS

For the Rub

2 dry chipotle peppers, seeded and minced

1 tablespoon dried oregano

1 tablespoon dried cilantro

1 tablespoon ground black pepper

2 teaspoons ground cumin

1 teaspoon onion powder

½ teaspoon dry mustard

Sea salt, to taste

For the Steak

1 tablespoon extra virgin olive oil

2 bone-in rib eyes (16 oz. each), about 1¼ to 1½ inches thick

1 Combine the rub ingredients and mix thoroughly. Rub a very thin layer of oil on both sides of the steaks and then generously apply the dry rub, firmly pressing it into the steaks. Let rest at room temperature for at least 1 hour.

2 A half hour before cooking, prepare your gas or charcoal grill to medium-high heat.

3 When the grill is ready, at about 400°F to 450°F with the coals lightly covered with ash, place the steaks on the grill and cook for about 6 to 7 minutes until blood begins to pool on the tops. When the steaks are charred, flip and cook for 4 to 5 more minutes for medium-rare and 5 to 6 more minutes for medium. The steaks should feel slightly firm if poked in the center.

4 Remove the steaks from the grill and transfer to a large cutting board. Let stand for 5 to 10 minutes, allowing the steaks to properly store their juices and flavor. Serve warm.

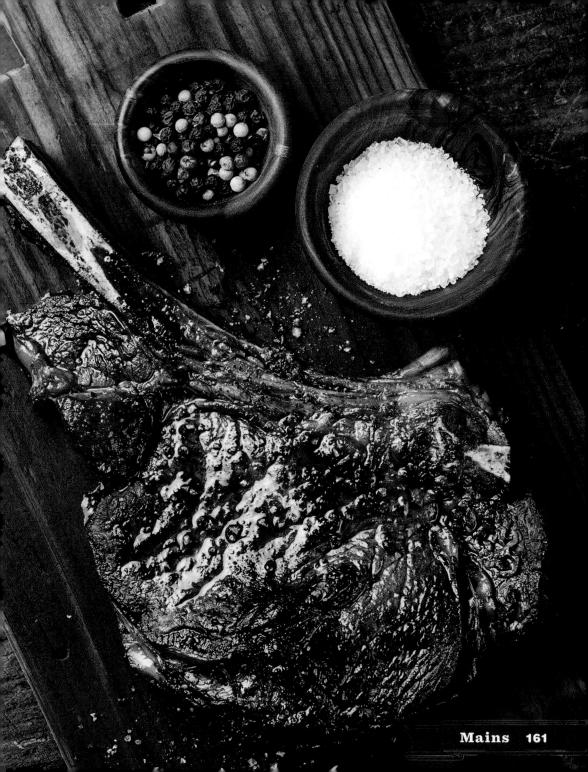

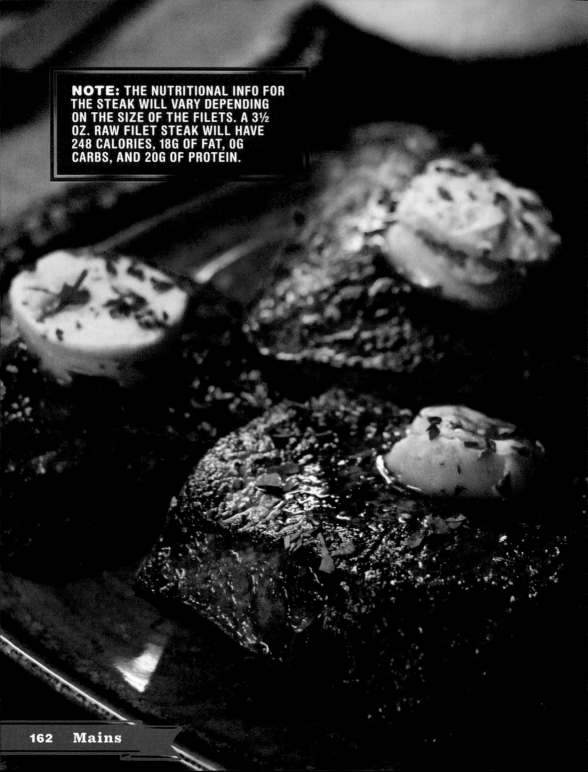

NOTE: THE NUTRITIONAL INFO FOR THE STEAK WILL VARY DEPENDING ON THE SIZE OF THE FILETS. A 3½ OZ. RAW FILET STEAK WILL HAVE 248 CALORIES, 18G OF FAT, 0G CARBS, AND 20G OF PROTEIN.

Tenderloin Steak with Herbed Butter

YIELD: 4 SERVINGS • PREP TIME: 10 MINUTES • COOK TIME: 15 MINUTES
NUTRITIONAL INFO (FOR THE HERB BUTTER): CALORIES: 113 • FAT: 12G •
NET CARBS: 1G • PROTEIN: 0G

The only thing that makes a perfectly cooked filet better is a dab of herb-infused butter.

1 Allow the butter to rest at room temperature until softened, or microwave until soft.

2 Combine parsley, garlic, pepper, and softened butter and mix well. Place herb-butter mixture into the fridge to firm up.

3 Season the steak with salt and pepper on both sides and heat the oil in a cast-iron skillet. Cook the steak for about 4 minutes on each side

4 Allow the steak to rest for 5 minutes, cut into filets, then top with a tablespoon of the herb butter and serve.

INGREDIENTS

4 tablespoons salted butter

2½ teaspoons parsley, chopped

2½ teaspoons garlic, minced

½ teaspoon black pepper

8¾ oz. beef tenderloin

Salt and pepper, to taste

1 teaspoon olive oil

Basil Pork Chops

YIELD: 4 SERVINGS • PREP TIME: 40 TO 50 MINUTES
COOK TIME: ABOUT 10 MINUTES
NUTRITIONAL INFO: CALORIES: 295 • FAT: 21G • NET CARBS: 1G • PROTEIN: 24G

The trick to cooking pork chops isn't in the seasoning, it all depends on how long you cook the meat. Pork chops tend to dry out very suddenly—if you have a meat thermometer on hand, check the internal temperature regularly until it reads 145°F, then remove from heat immediately.

INGREDIENTS

2 garlic cloves, minced

1 cup fresh basil leaves, minced

2 tablespoons lemon juice

2 tablespoons extra virgin olive oil

Salt and pepper, to taste

4 pork loin chops, bone-in

1 In a small bowl, combine the garlic, basil, lemon juice, oil, salt, and pepper. Spread over the pork chops and marinate for 30 to 45 minutes. Preheat your grill to medium heat while you wait.

2 Grill over medium heat for about 4 minutes on each side, or until the pork chops are tender.

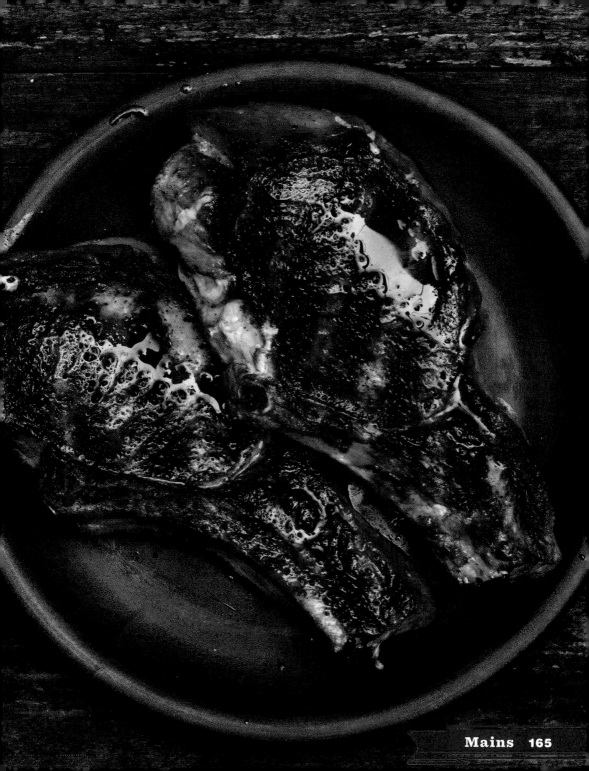

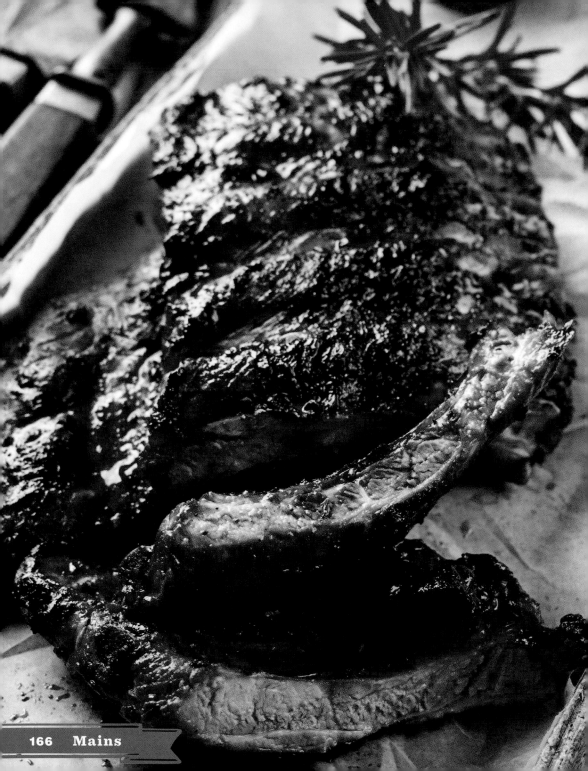

Chili and Cayenne Spareribs

YIELD: 6 SERVINGS • PREP TIME: 10 MINUTES • COOK TIME: 8 TO 10 HOURS
NUTRITIONAL INFO: CALORIES: 402 • FAT: 34G • NET CARBS: 1G • PROTEIN: 20G

As you make the spicy sauce with the tomatoes, consider varying the flavor by using more or less of the listed spices, or even adding something else you like. Just make sure not to overdo the cinnamon.

1 Put the oil in a baking dish. Put the ribs in the dish and toss to coat with oil. Sprinkle the oiled ribs with cayenne, salt, and pepper and place in the slow cooker.

2 In a bowl, combine the tomatoes, water, cumin, cinnamon, ancho chili powder, and garlic powder. Pour over ribs, then cover and cook on Low for 8 to 10 hours.

3 Skim fat off the top of the dish, finish the ribs on the grill if you want them crispy on the outside, and serve with sauce on the side.

INGREDIENTS

2 tablespoons extra virgin olive oil

3 lbs. country-style thick-cut spareribs

1 teaspoon cayenne pepper

Salt and pepper, to taste

2 tomatoes, pureed

Water, enough to make sauce without it becoming too thin

1 teaspoon cumin

½ teaspoon cinnamon

½ teaspoon ancho chili powder

½ teaspoon garlic powder

Grilled and Roasted Pork Loin

YIELD: 5 TO 6 SERVINGS • PREP TIME: 25 MINUTES • COOK TIME: 1 HOUR
NUTRITIONAL INFO: CALORIES: 365 • FAT: 21G • NET CARBS: 0G • PROTEIN: 43G

For any oven-to-grill recipe, avoid using cookware that has a plastic, wood, or synthetic handle. It is best if the pan has rounded sides high enough to prevent the oil from spilling or flaring up when basting. Top each serving with a tablespoon of butter to add fat macros to this dish.

INGREDIENTS

5 tablespoons extra virgin olive oil

1 or 2 sprigs fresh rosemary

2¼-pound. pork loin

Salt and pepper, to taste

1 Fire up the grill and allow the coals to settle into a temperature of about 350°F. While the grill is heating, sauté the oil and rosemary in a cast-iron skillet or another high heat–friendly pan. Be sure the pan is oven-and-grill friendly, as it will be placed directly onto the grill.

2 After the oil and rosemary have been thoroughly heated and the flavors of the sprigs are infused throughout the oil (about 10 to 12 minutes), rub the pork loin with the salt and pepper, and place the pork loin into the pan, turning it so the entire loin is covered with the heated oil.

3 Baste for 5 to 10 minutes while cooking over medium heat until the loin begins to brown. Once the grill has reached the desired temperature, move the entire pan to the grill grate.

4 Cover the grill and allow the pork to cook for 45 minutes, turning and basting the pork occasionally so all sides are thoroughly browned.

5 At about 45 minutes, remove the pork loin from the pan and place directly on the grill. Continue to baste the pork loin using the infused oil from the pan, turning the loin so the entire roast spends some time on of the grill. Baste and turn for an additional 15 or so minutes or until the roast meets your desired temperature.

6 Remove from fire and let the loin rest for 10 to 12 minutes. Carve and serve with a side of your choice.

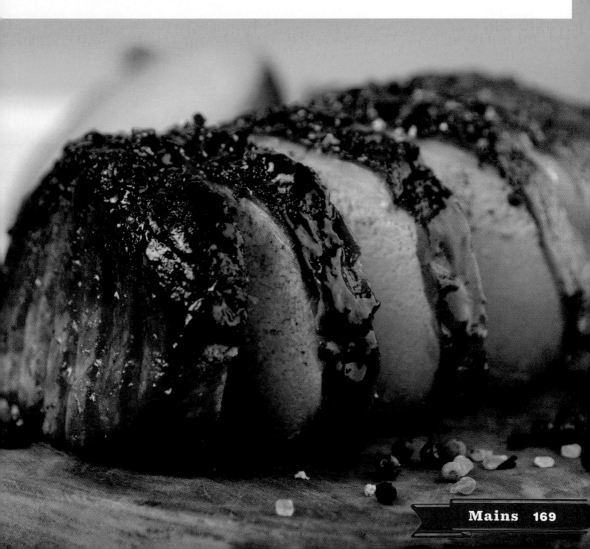

Pork Chili Fry

YIELD: 1 SERVING • PREP TIME: 10 MINUTES • COOK TIME: 10 MINUTES
NUTRITIONAL INFO: CALORIES: 394 • FAT: 21G • NET CARBS: 5G • PROTEIN: 43G

A delicious fusion dish that borrows a bit from India and a bit from China.

INGREDIENTS

7 oz. pork tenderloin

Salt and pepper, to taste

1 tablespoon vegetable oil

1 spring onion, chopped, white and green sections separated

1 teaspoon garlic, chopped

1 teaspoon ginger, chopped

¼ cup green peppers, chopped

2 green chili peppers, sliced (remove seeds to reduce spice)

1 teaspoon soy sauce

1 teaspoon black vinegar

1 Chop the pork tenderloin into bite-size pieces and season with salt and pepper.

2 Heat the oil in a wok or large pan and fry the spring onion whites, garlic, and ginger until the garlic starts to brown.

3 Add in the pork and fry until it starts to brown. Then, add in the peppers, soy sauce, and vinegar. Cook until pork is cooked through.

4 Remove wok from heat, garnish with spring onion greens, and serve.

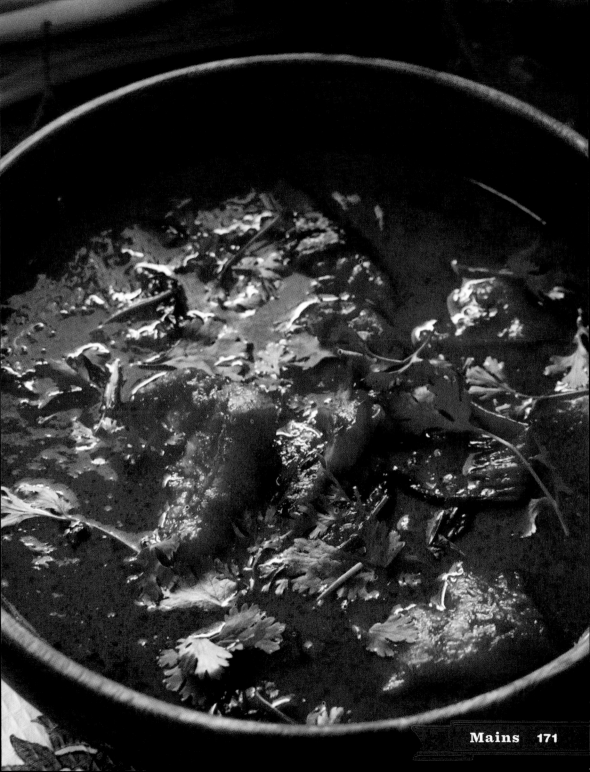

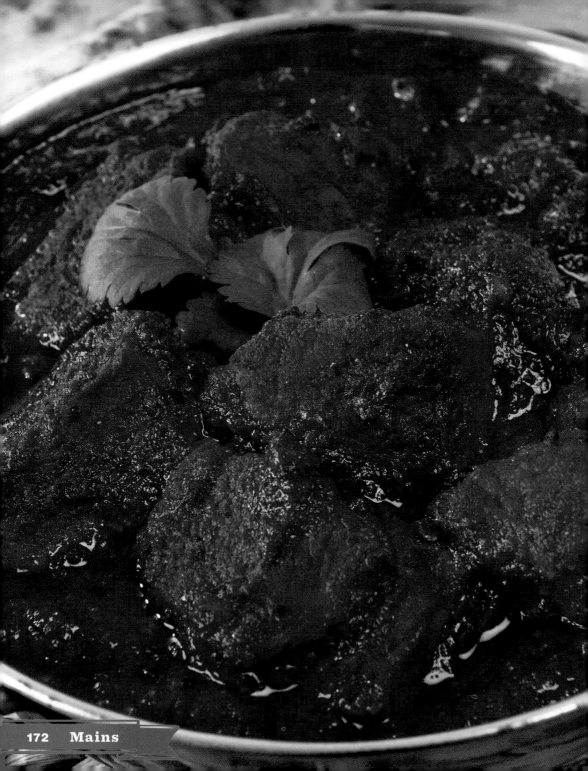

Pork Vindaloo

YIELD: 6 SERVINGS • PREP TIME: 5 MINUTES • COOK TIME: ABOUT 4 TO 8 HOURS
NUTRITIONAL INFO: CALORIES: 590 • FAT: 41G • NET CARBS: 7G • PROTEIN: 46G

The whole cloves of garlic in this recipe are a treat to eat. The garlic gets soft, loses its bite, and becomes infused with the other spices.

1 Heat oil in a skillet over medium-high heat and add slices of onions. Cook, stirring frequently, for about 3 minutes, until onions are translucent.

2 Add tomatoes, chilies, turmeric, coriander, garam masala, and cinnamon, stirring constantly until the onions, tomatoes, and chilies are coated with the spices. Remove from heat.

3 Put the pork into the slow cooker, and add the onion, chili, and tomato spice mixture. Add the garlic cloves, apple cider vinegar, ginger, and dry mustard and stir well. Pour the water over the pork mixture. Cover and cook on Low for 6 to 8 hours or on High for 4 to 5 hours.

INGREDIENTS

2 tablespoons extra virgin olive oil

1 large onion, sliced thin

16 oz. fresh tomatoes, finely chopped

6 chilies, such as jalapeños, habaneros, or a combination, seeded and sliced

1 teaspoon turmeric

1 teaspoon ground coriander

1½ teaspoons garam masala

½ teaspoon cinnamon

2½-pound. pork butt, trimmed and cut into cubes

10 garlic cloves, peeled

2 tablespoons apple cider vinegar

2 tablespoons fresh ginger, grated

1 teaspoon dry mustard powder

2 cups water

Rosemary-Braised Pork

YIELD: 6 SERVINGS • PREP TIME: 10 MINUTES • COOK TIME: ABOUT 2½ HOURS
NUTRITIONAL INFO: CALORIES: 505 • FAT: 39G • NET CARBS: 3G • PROTEIN: 42G

For a summery variation, consider substituting the 2 sprigs of rosemary with 3 tablespoons freshly chopped dill.

INGREDIENTS

2 sprigs rosemary, needles removed

2¼-pound boneless pork loin

8 tablespoons extra virgin olive oil

1 garlic clove, crushed

½ onion, chopped

¾ cup white wine

1 tablespoon white vinegar

Salt and pepper, to taste

1 Preheat your grill to medium heat. To enhance the flavor and to prevent the rosemary from searing completely off during the cooking process, push the rosemary needles into the meat. This will help infuse the flavor throughout the pork. Leave a little bit of each rosemary sprig sticking out to catch and burn from the flame; this adds to the flavor.

2 Brush and coat the roast with oil. Place the roast into a deep sauté pan that can withstand the direct heat of the grill. Place the pan on the grill and place the remaining oil into the pan, turning and cooking the pork evenly on all sides until it reaches a lovely golden brown.

3 Add the garlic, onion, and wine and let the meat and seasoning cook together for about an hour. If you can control the temperature of the grill, bring the heat down so everything may simmer together for 1½ hours.

4 Just before the pork appears to be done, remove it from the pan and place it directly on the grill to char the exterior to your preference.

5 Remove the roast from the grill, and let it stand for 10 to 12 minutes. Slice thin before serving. Add the white vinegar, salt, pepper to the juices and use as a light gravy.

Thai-Style Fried Rice

YIELD: 4 SERVINGS • PREP TIME: 10 MINUTES • COOK TIME: 5 MINUTES
NUTRITIONAL INFO: CALORIES: 321 • FAT: 26G • NET CARBS: 3G • PROTEIN: 14G

A delicious pork fried rice, flavored with the spices of Thai green curry.

INGREDIENTS

1 tablespoon coconut oil

2¼ tablespoons Thai green curry paste

8¾ oz. ground pork

Salt, to taste

1 spring onion, chopped, white and green sections separated

¾ cup coconut milk

17½ oz. cooked Riced Cauliflower (see page 81)

1 Heat coconut oil in a wok and add the curry paste, frying until fragrant.

2 Add the pork, season with salt, and cook for 2 minutes. Add in the spring onion whites and cook for 30 seconds, then add the coconut milk.

3 Simmer for 2 minutes. Taste and adjust seasoning as desired.

4 Fold in Riced Cauliflower and cook until well mixed and the coconut milk has soaked into the rice. Garnish with the spring onion greens and serve.

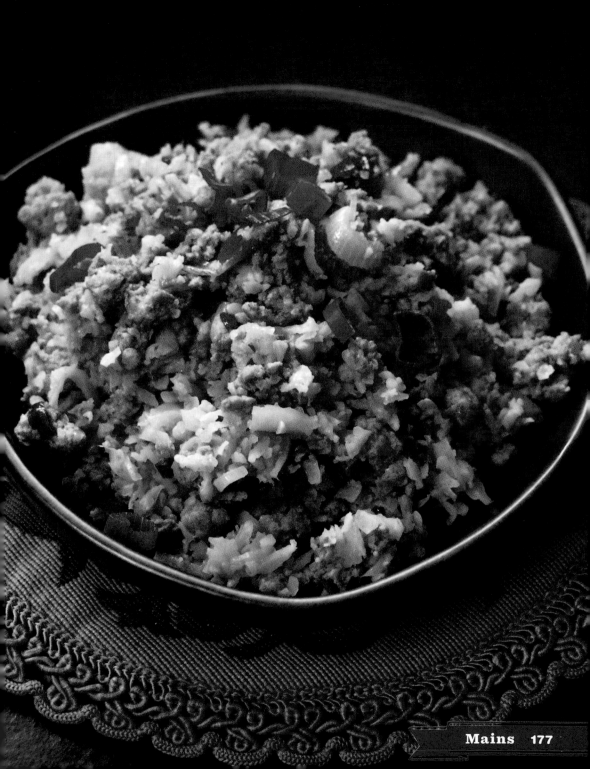

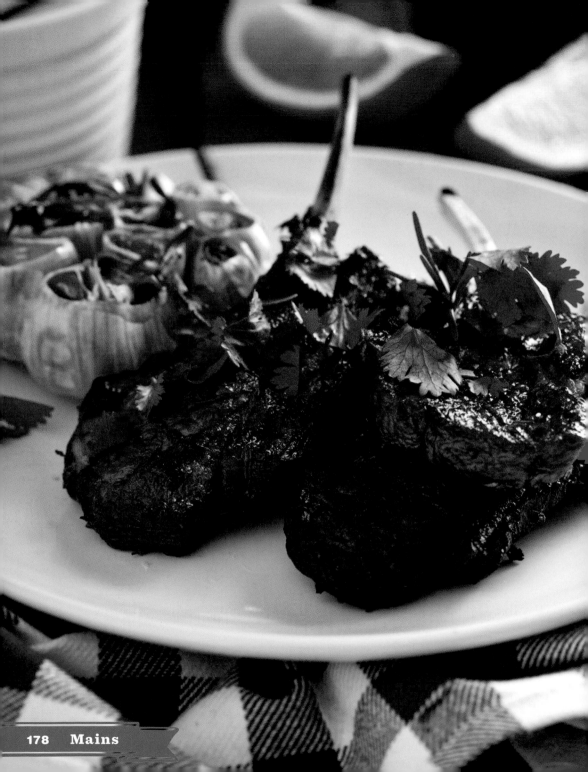

Broiled Rosemary and Lemon Lamb Chops

YIELD: 4 SERVINGS • PREP TIME: 10 MINUTES • COOK TIME: 5 MINUTES
NUTRITIONAL INFO: CALORIES: 356 • FAT: 22G • NET CARBS: 3G • PROTEIN: 33G

Lamb chops are an indulgence, for sure, so if you're going to splurge, be sure to follow this recipe when preparing them. The rosemary, garlic, and lemon bring out the earthy goodness of the chops.

1 Preheat the broiler to high. Position a rack to be about 5 to 7 inches away from the heat. Put the skillet in the oven so it gets hot.

2 In a bowl, combine the lemon juice and rosemary. Press the garlic into the mix and season with salt and pepper. Using your hands, rub the chops in the mix, being sure to coat both sides evenly. Put the chops on a platter.

3 When the skillet is hot, take it out and position the chops in it so they fit. Return to the rack under the broiler and cook for about 5 minutes. Since the skillet is already hot, the lamb cooks on both sides at once.

4 Remove from the oven, let rest for a minute, and serve.

INGREDIENTS

4 tablespoons lemon juice

2 tablespoons fresh rosemary leaves, chopped

2 garlic cloves, pressed

Salt and pepper, to taste

8 lamb chops (approx. 24 oz. with bone in)

Grilled Garlic-Herb Rack of Lamb

YIELD: 5 TO 6 SERVINGS • PREP TIME: 12 HOURS 10 MINUTES
COOK TIME: 10 MINUTES
NUTRITIONAL INFO: CALORIES: 323 • FAT: 20G • NET CARBS: 3G • PROTEIN: 31G

Because a rack of lamb is very delicate, be sure to give it the time to marinate overnight.

INGREDIENTS

For the Rack of Lamb

2 tablespoons extra virgin olive oil

2 garlic cloves, finely chopped

1 teaspoon lemon zest

2 8-rib racks of lamb (approx. 1 lb. each)

Salt and pepper, to taste

For the Garlic-Herb Crust

4 garlic cloves, finely chopped

½ small shallot, finely chopped

¼ cup flat-leaf parsley, coarsely chopped

2 tablespoons rosemary, finely chopped

1 tablespoon thyme, finely chopped

Salt and pepper, to taste

1 The night before grilling, combine the oil, garlic, and lemon zest in a large resealable plastic bag. Pat dry the racks of lamb, and then season them with salt and pepper, kneading the pepper and salt deeply into the meaty sections of the lamb. Add the racks of lamb into plastic bag and place in the refrigerator. Let marinate overnight.

2 An hour and a half before grilling, remove the racks of lamb from the refrigerator and let rest, uncovered and at room temperature.

3 A half hour before grilling, prepare your gas or charcoal grill to medium heat.

4 While the grill heats, combine all of the ingredients for the crust in a small bowl. Next, take the racks of lamb and generously apply the crust ingredients to it, being sure to apply the majority of the crust on the meaty side of the rack.

5 When the grill is ready, at about 400°F with the coals are lightly covered with ash, place the meaty side of the racks of lamb on the grill and cook for about 3 to 4 minutes. When the crusts are browned, flip the racks of lamb and grill for another 5 minutes for medium-rare.

6 Transfer the racks of lamb from the grill to a large carving board and let rest for about 10 minutes before slicing between the ribs. Serve warm.

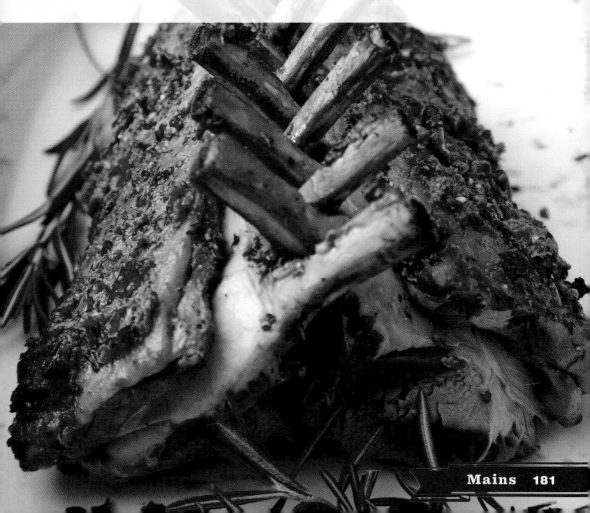

Mint Lamb Kebabs

YIELD: 8 TO 10 SERVINGS • PREP TIME: 4 TO 16 HOURS
COOK TIME: 15 TO 20 MINUTES
NUTRITIONAL INFO: CALORIES: 390 • FAT: 33G • NET CARBS: 2G • PROTEIN: 20G

The mint chimichurri adds the perfect kick of flavor to take these simple lamb kebabs over the top.

INGREDIENTS

Tools

24 skewers

For the Lamb

2 lbs. lamb, cut into 1½-inch cubes

Salt and pepper, to taste

4 tablespoons extra virgin olive oil

4 garlic cloves, crushed

2 teaspoons rosemary, finely chopped

1 teaspoon ground cumin

1 red onion, cut into square pieces

1 red pepper, cut into square pieces

For the Mint Chimichurri

2 garlic cloves

2 cups flat-leaf parsley

2 cups mint leaves

1 small shallot

Juice of ¼ small lime

4 tablespoons red wine vinegar

½ cup extra virgin olive oil

Salt and pepper, to taste

1 The night before you plan to grill, season the lamb cubes with salt and pepper. Set aside.

2 Next, in a large resealable plastic bag (if you need two, divide recipe between both bags), combine the remaining ingredients except for the onion and pepper. Add the lamb cubes to the bag and then transfer to the refrigerator, letting the meat marinate from 4 hours to overnight, the longer the better.

3 An hour and a half before grilling, remove the lamb from the refrigerator and let rest, uncovered and outside of the marinade, at room temperature.

4 To make the mint chimichurri, in a small food processor, puree the garlic, parsley, mint, shallot, lime juice, and vinegar. Slowly add the olive oil, and then remove the sauce from the processor. Season with salt and pepper, cover, and set aside.

5 A half hour before grilling, prepare your gas or charcoal grill to medium-high heat.

6 Pierce about four lamb cubes with each bamboo skewer, making sure to align the pieces of onion and pepper in between each cube.

7 When the grill is ready, at about 450°F with the coals lightly covered with ash, place the skewers on the grill and cook for about 15 to 20 minutes. Transfer the kebabs to a large carving board and let them rest for 5 minutes before serving with the mint chimichurri.

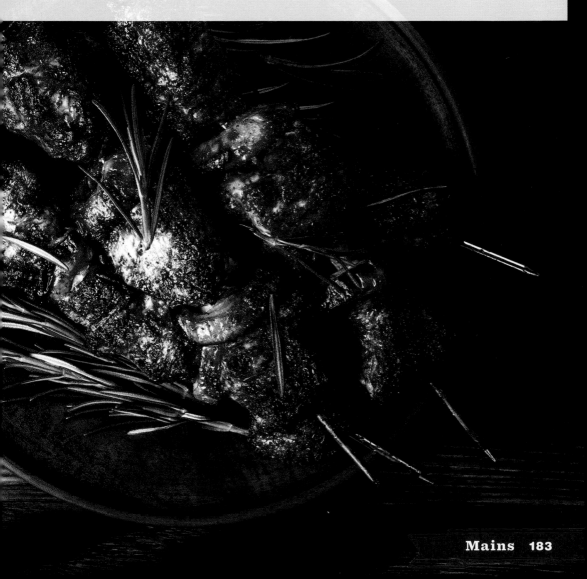

Paprika Lamb Chops

YIELD: 4 SERVINGS • PREP TIME: 1 HOUR 15 MINUTES • COOK TIME: 15 MINUTES
NUTRITIONAL INFO: CALORIES: 706 • FAT: 51G • NET CARBS: 0G • PROTEIN: 48G

The paprika-salt rub works well on almost anything, including beef, poultry, vegetables, and most fish.

INGREDIENTS

12 lamb rib chops, each about 1-inch thick (approx. 36 oz.)

2 tablespoons extra virgin olive oil

2 tablespoons smoked paprika

1 tablespoon cumin seeds

2 teaspoons coriander seeds

½ teaspoon cayenne pepper

Salt and pepper, to taste

1 An hour before grilling, brush the lamb rib chops with oil and let stand at room temperature.

2 In a small bowl, mix together the remaining ingredients to make a paprika-salt rub. Using your hands, generously apply the rub to the lamb rib chops.

3 Prepare your gas or charcoal grill to medium-high heat. When the grill is ready, at about 400°F to 450°F with the coals lightly covered with ash, place the lamb rib chops on the grill and cook for about 4 minutes or until the spices have browned. Turn the chops and cook for another 3 to 4 minutes for medium-rare, 4 to 5 minutes for medium.

4 Transfer the lamb rib chops to a large carving board and let stand for 5 minutes before serving.

Slow Cooker Leg of Lamb

YIELD: 8 SERVINGS • PREP TIME: 10 MINUTES • COOK TIME: 6 TO 8 HOURS
NUTRITIONAL INFO: CALORIES: 505 • FAT: 34G • NET CARBS: 1G • PROTEIN: 48G

Serve the lamb with a lively sugar-free mint sauce. Make it by chopping together ½ cup fresh mint leaves and ½ cup fresh parsley leaves. Stir in about ½ cup oil, salt and pepper to taste, and a squeeze or so of fresh lemon juice. If you feel it needs some sweetening, stir in a teaspoon of stevia.

1 Using your hands, rub the oil all over the leg of lamb. Put the lamb in the slow cooker and sprinkle it all over with the salt, pepper, rosemary, mint, and garlic, rubbing the spices onto the meat.

2 Cover and cook on Low for 6 to 8 hours. Do not cook on High.

3 If desired with additional salt and pepper and serve.

INGREDIENTS

1 bone-in leg of lamb (shank removed)

1 tablespoon extra virgin olive oil

½ teaspoon salt

½ teaspoon freshly ground black pepper

1 teaspoon fresh rosemary, chopped

1 teaspoon fresh mint, chopped

3 garlic cloves, minced

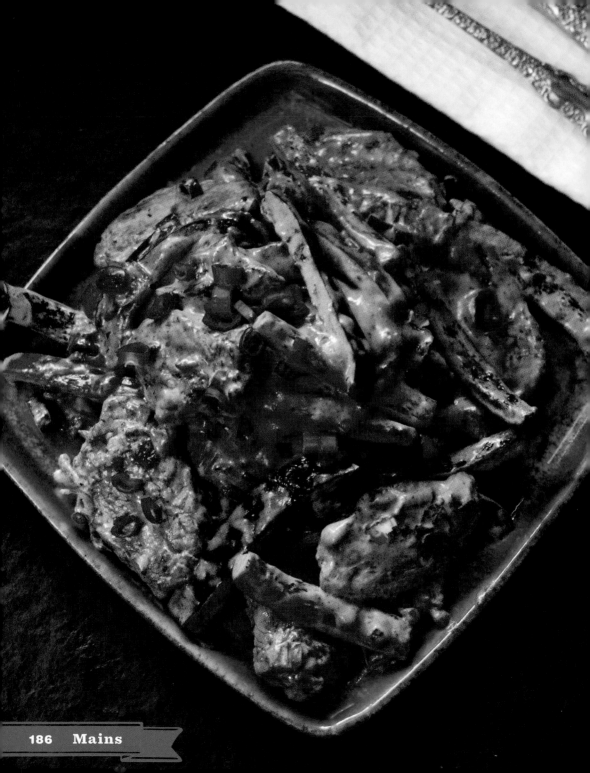

Creamy Pork Tenderloin

YIELD: 1 SERVING • PREP TIME: 5 MINUTES • COOK TIME: 15 MINUTES
NUTRITIONAL INFO: CALORIES: 602 • FAT: 42G • NET CARBS: 5G • PROTEIN: 49G

Pan-seared pork loin pairs perfectly with this rich creamy sauce.

1 Chop and marinate the pork with half the olive oil, salt, pepper, and the Parmesan cheese and let stand for 5 minutes.

2 Heat the remaining olive oil in a frying pan and cook the pork on high heat for about 1 to 2 minutes and then remove from the pan.

3 Using the same pan, cook the butter, garlic, peppers, and white part of spring onions for 3 to 4 minutes.

4 Once the peppers have softened add in the cream along with the pork and cook for 2 minutes.

5 Garnish with the spring onion greens and serve.

INGREDIENTS

7 oz. pork tenderloin

1 tablespoon olive oil

Salt and pepper, to taste

1 tablespoon Parmesan cheese

1 teaspoon butter

2 garlic cloves, minced

¾ oz. red and yellow bell peppers

1½ tablespoons spring onion, chopped, white and green sections separated

4 tablespoons heavy cream

Basil and Chili Chicken Breasts

BASIL CHICKEN BREASTS: YIELD: 4 SERVINGS • PREP TIME: 12½ TO 14 HOURS •
COOK TIME: 30 MINUTES
NUTRITIONAL INFO (FOR CHICKEN BREASTS): CALORIES: 172 • FAT: 7G •
NET CARBS: 4G • PROTEIN: 23G
CHILI OIL YIELD: 12 SERVINGS
NUTRITIONAL INFO (FOR CHILI OIL): CALORIES: 120 • FAT: 14G •
NET CARBS: 0G • PROTEIN: 0G

If the chili oil is a little intense when added directly to the chicken, you can always serve it on the side for a milder meal.

INGREDIENTS

For the Chili Oil

2 chili peppers of your choice

¾ cup extra virgin olive oil

1 garlic clove, crushed

1 teaspoon ground coriander

For the Chicken

2 cups fresh basil leaves

3 spring onions, chopped

2 garlic cloves

1 chili pepper of your choice, stemmed and coarsely chopped

¼ to ½ cup extra virgin olive oil

4 skin-on, boneless chicken breasts (4 oz. each)

Salt and pepper, to taste

1 Add chili peppers into a small saucepan over medium-high heat. Lightly toast until the skin is blackened, about 3 to 4 minutes. Remove the chili peppers and set aside. Next, add the oil to the saucepan and heat. Mix in garlic and coriander and cook for 4 to 5 minutes. Then, add the chilies and cook for 4 more minutes. Remove and let rest overnight. You can store the oil up to 4 months. Keep in mind that the longer the chilies infuse into the oil, the hotter it will be.

2 Mix the basil leaves, spring onions, garlic, and chili pepper in a large bowl, and then add oil. Add the chicken breasts into the marinade and place in the refrigerator. Let soak for at least 4 hours or overnight.

3 Remove the chili oil from the refrigerator and set aside. Transfer the chicken from the marinade to a large cutting board and let rest at room temperature for 30 minutes to 1 hour.

4 Prepare your gas or charcoal grill to medium-high heat.

5 When the grill is ready, at about 400°F to 450°F with the coals lightly covered with ash, place the chicken on the grill and cook for about 7 minutes. Flip and grill for another 5 to 6 minutes until finished; they should feel springy if poked.

6 Remove and let rest for 5 minutes. Serve warm with a drizzle of chili oil and season with salt and pepper.

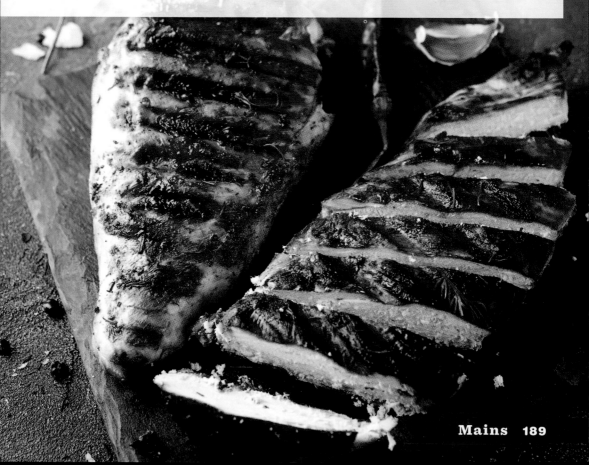

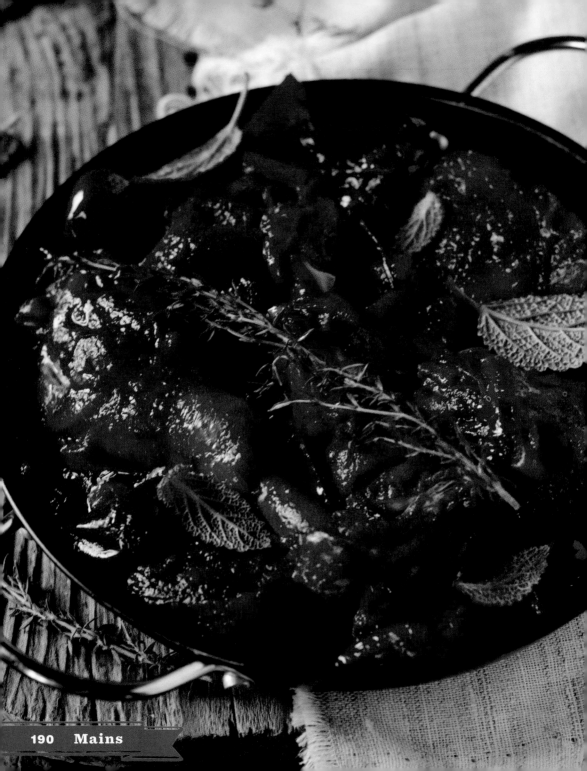

Chicken Cacciatore

YIELD: 6 SERVINGS • PREP TIME: 10 MINUTES • COOK TIME: ABOUT 3 TO 8 HOURS

NUTRITIONAL INFO: CALORIES: 263 • FAT: 13G • NET CARBS: 5G • PROTEIN: 27G

This meal is even better the second day. Just make sure to serve it over some Riced Cauliflower (page 81).

1 Rinse the chicken and pat dry with paper towels. Preheat the oven broiler. Then, line a broiler pan with heavy-duty aluminum foil. Broil chicken pieces for 3 minutes per side, or until browned. Transfer pieces to the slow cooker.

2 Heat oil in a large skillet over medium-high heat. Add onion, garlic, and mushrooms and cook, stirring frequently, for 5 minutes, or until mushrooms begin to soften. Scrape mixture into the slow cooker.

3 Add the tomatoes and their juices, wine, thyme, sage, and rosemary to the slow cooker, and stir well. Cook on Low for 6 to 8 hours or on High for 3 to 4 hours, or until chicken is cooked through, tender, and no longer pink. Season with salt and pepper and serve.

INGREDIENTS

6 chicken breasts, skin removed (approx. 24 oz.)

¼ cup extra virgin olive oil

1 large onion, halved and thinly sliced

2 garlic cloves, minced

1 lb. cremini mushrooms, wiped with a damp paper towel, trimmed, and sliced

1 (14 oz.) can diced tomatoes, with their juices

½ cup dry white wine

1 tablespoon fresh thyme

1 tablespoon fresh sage, chopped

1 tablespoon fresh rosemary, chopped

Salt and pepper, to taste

Chicken Fried Rice

YIELD: 2 SERVINGS • PREP TIME: 15 MINUTES • COOK TIME: 10 MINUTES
NUTRITIONAL INFO: CALORIES: 385 • FAT: 26G • NET CARBS: 6G • PROTEIN: 29G

You won't miss traditional rice with this Riced Cauliflower stir fry.

INGREDIENTS

2 eggs

Salt and pepper, to taste

2 tablespoons olive oil

4 teaspoons spring onion, chopped, white and green sections separated

1 garlic clove, chopped

5 oz. boneless chicken thighs, cut into small pieces

½ cup white mushrooms, sliced

¼ cup green bell peppers, sliced

10½ oz. cooked Riced Cauliflower (see page 81)

1 tablespoon soy sauce

1 tablespoon white vinegar

1 Beat the eggs and season with salt and pepper.

2 Heat 1 tablespoon of oil in a pan, then add the eggs and quickly scramble them.

3 In a wok, heat 1 tablespoon of oil and fry the spring onion whites, garlic, and chicken, and season with salt and pepper. Add in the mushrooms and green peppers and cook until tender.

4 Combine the Riced Cauliflower and scrambled eggs with chicken and vegetables. Add in the soy sauce and vinegar and cook for 2 more minutes.

5 Garnish with spring onion greens and serve.

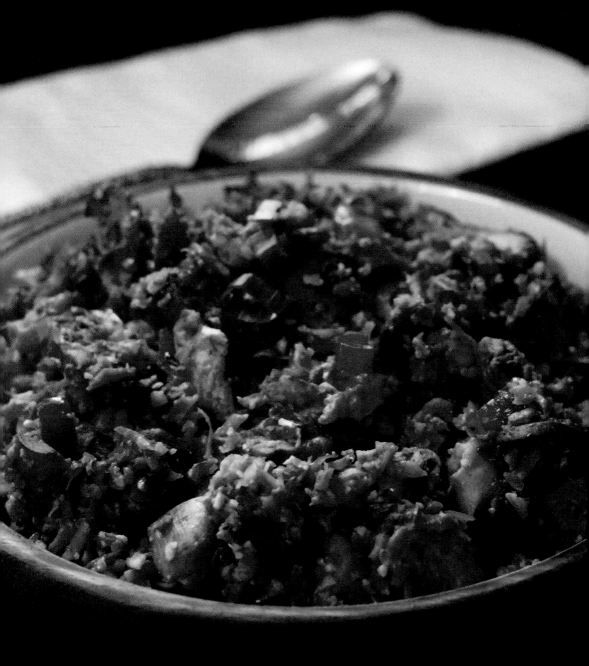

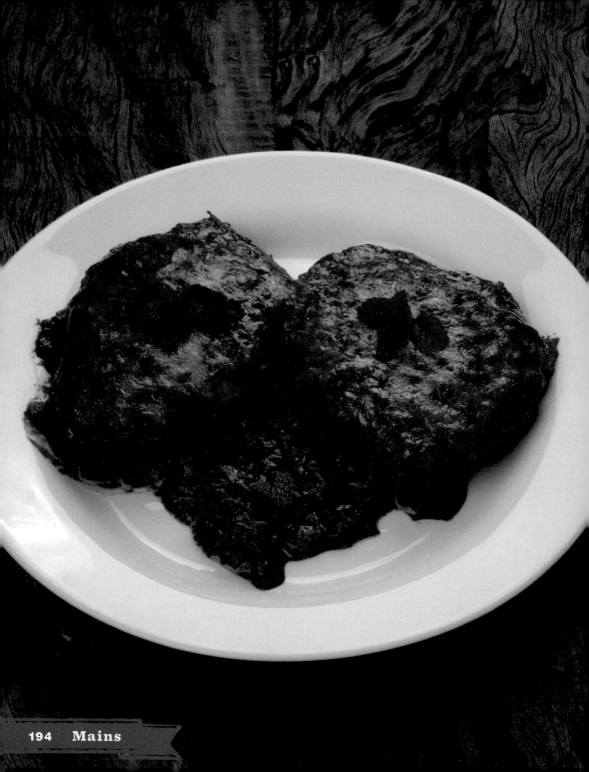

Chicken Parmigiana

YIELD: 4 SERVINGS • PREP TIME: 5 MINUTES • COOK TIME: 4½ TO 7 HOURS
NUTRITIONAL INFO: CALORIES: 388 • FAT: 22G • NET CARBS: 4G • PROTEIN: 45G

Rather than sprinkle the meat with the seasonings, you can add them to your spaghetti sauce before pouring it on the chicken. You can also try a marinara sauce that has basil or red peppers, so long as there is no sugar added.

1 Place the chicken breasts in the slow cooker. Sprinkle with garlic powder, salt, pepper, Italian seasoning, and Parmesan cheese. Pour the spaghetti sauce over the meat.

2 Cover and cook on Low for 6 hours or on High for 4 hours.

3 Uncover and top the chicken with the mozzarella cheese. Cover and continue to cook on Low for another hour or on High for another 30 minutes.

INGREDIENTS

4 boneless, skinless chicken breasts (approx. 16 oz.)

1 teaspoon garlic powder

Salt and pepper, to taste

1 teaspoon Italian seasoning mix

½ cup Parmesan cheese, grated

1 cup no-sugar spaghetti sauce (Prego and Classico both make these)

2 cups shredded mozzarella cheese

Grilled Chicken Breast with Sesame Seeds and Ginger

YIELD: 4 SERVINGS • PREP TIME: 40 MINUTES • COOK TIME: 15 MINUTES
NUTRITIONAL INFO: CALORIES: 325 • FAT: 16G • NET CARBS: 2G • PROTEIN: 45G

The combination of sesame seeds and ginger is hard to beat, especially with the added hint of smokiness from the grill.

INGREDIENTS

2 tablespoons, plus ½ teaspoon extra virgin olive oil

1- to 2-inch piece ginger, peeled and sliced

2 spring onions, finely chopped

2 garlic cloves, minced

Juice of ½ small lemon

4 boneless chicken breasts (2 lbs. total)

Salt and pepper, to taste

3 tablespoons sesame seeds

1 Heat 2 tablespoons of the oil in a small skillet over medium-high heat. Once hot, add the ginger, spring onions, garlic, and lemon juice and sauté for about 2 to 3 minutes, or until the onions are translucent and the garlic is crisp but not browned. Remove from heat and transfer to a small bowl.

2 Rub the chicken breasts with salt and pepper and put them in a resealable plastic bag. Add the ginger-and-onion mixture and press around the chicken breasts. Seal and let rest at room temperature for 30 minutes.

3 Prepare your gas or charcoal grill to medium-high heat.

4 In a small dish, mix ½ teaspoon oil with sesame seeds. Set aside.

5 When the grill is ready, about 400°F to 450°F with the coals lightly covered with ash, place the chicken on the grill and sprinkle the tops with half of the oiled sesame seeds. Grill the chicken breasts for about 7 minutes. Flip and season with the remaining sesame seeds, and then grill for 5 to 6 more minutes. When finished, they should feel springy if poked.

6 Remove and let rest for 5 minutes. Serve warm.

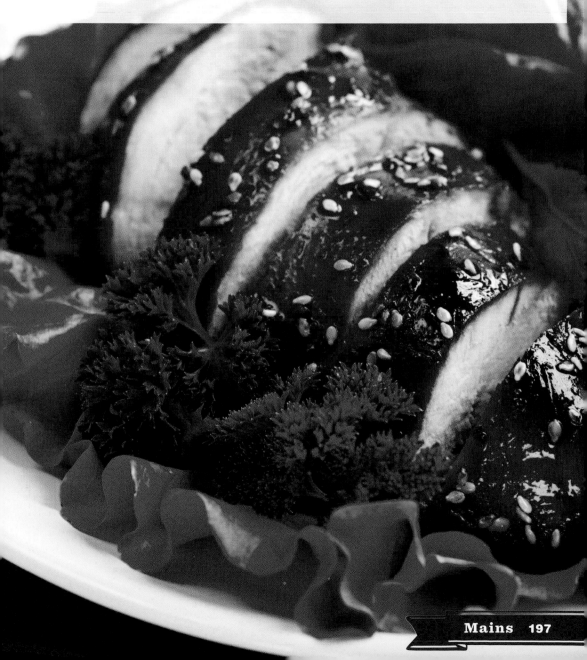

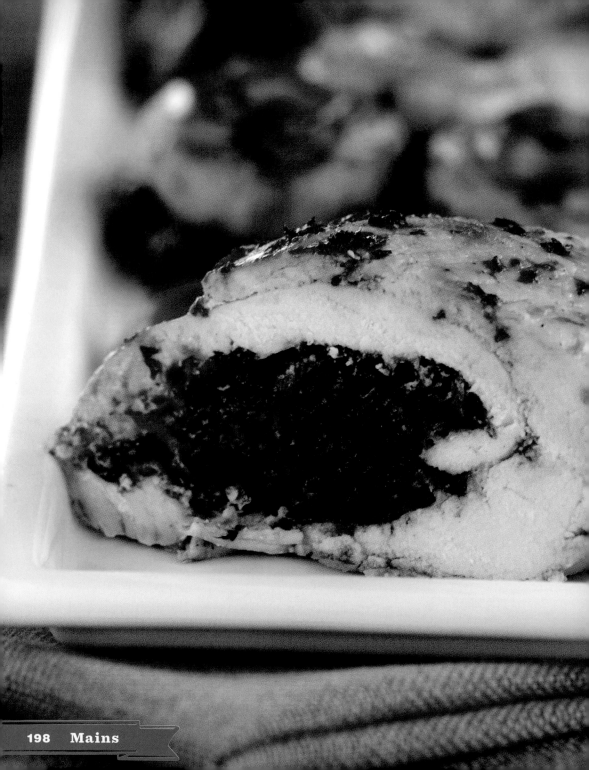

Kale and Cheese-Stuffed Chicken Breasts

YIELD: 4 SERVINGS • PREP TIME: 15 MINUTES • COOK TIME: 5 TO 8 HOURS
NUTRITIONAL INFO: CALORIES: 389 • FAT: 22G • NET CARBS: 3G • PROTEIN: 38G

To add even more protein to this recipe, cook 4 strips of bacon in the microwave until crispy, and add one to each breast before rolling them up.

1 The breasts should be on the thin side so they roll up easily. If they're thicker than ½- to ¼-inch, put them between pieces of waxed paper and use a meat mallet to pound them thin.

2 Sprinkle salt, pepper, oregano, onion powder, and cayenne on both sides of the chicken. Put a layer of chopped kale in the center of each breast, lay a strip or so of cheese to cover it, and then top with additional kale. Roll the breasts up tightly and secure with kitchen twine.

3 Lay the rolls in the slow cooker. Add the wine. Cover and cook on Low for 6 to 8 hours, or on High for about 5 hours, until the juices run clear and the cheese is melted. If you want to "crisp" the outside, transfer the rolls to a foil-lined baking sheet and put them under the broiler for a few minutes.

TOOLS
Kitchen twine

INGREDIENTS
4 boneless, skinless chicken breasts (approx. 16 oz. total)

Salt and pepper, to taste

¼ teaspoon dried oregano

½ teaspoon onion powder

½ teaspoon cayenne pepper

2 cups kale leaves, chopped

16 oz. cheddar cheese, cut into thick strips

½ cup dry white wine

Lemon and Garlic Grilled Chicken

YIELD: 4 TO 5 SERVINGS • PREP TIME: 25 MINUTES • COOK TIME: 1 HOUR
NUTRITIONAL INFO (FOR BREASTS): CALORIES: 228 • FAT: 9G •
NET CARBS: 0G • PROTEIN: 35G
NUTRITIONAL INFO (FOR DRUMSTICKS AND THIGHS): CALORIES: 310 •
FAT: 18G • NET CARBS: 0G • PROTEIN: 34G

Before filling the chicken's cavity with the garlic, thyme, and rosemary, heavily rinse the cavity with a couple cups of orange juice and a dash of salt to really up the flavor and wow your guests.

1 Prepare your gas or charcoal grill to medium heat.

2 Place the chicken into a large roasting pan and season its cavity generously with salt and pepper. Take 5 of the lemon halves and put them into the cavity, gently squeezing them while doing so. Then, grab the remaining lemon half and rub it across the chicken, squeezing it lightly so that its juices seep into the chicken. Discard this half. Fill the cavity with the garlic, thyme, and rosemary, and tie the legs together with the butcher's twine. Let rest for 15 minutes.

3 Take 4 tablespoons of extra virgin olive oil and massage it over the chicken's skin. Season the outside with additional pepper and salt.

4 When the grill is ready, at about 400°F with the coals lightly covered with ash, place the chicken on the grill, breast

TOOLS

1 to 2 feet
kitchen twine

INGREDIENTS

4- to 5-lb. chicken

Salt and pepper,
to taste

3 lemons, halved

1 garlic bulb,
halved

1 bunch thyme

1 bunch rosemary

5 tablespoons
extra virgin
olive oil

side up. Cover the grill and cook for about 40 minutes. Before flipping, brush the top of the chicken with the remaining tablespoon of oil. Turn and cook for about 15 more minutes until the skin is crisp and a meat thermometer inserted into the thickest part of the thigh reads 165°F.

5 Remove from grill and place on a large carving board. Let the chicken rest for 10 minutes before carving.

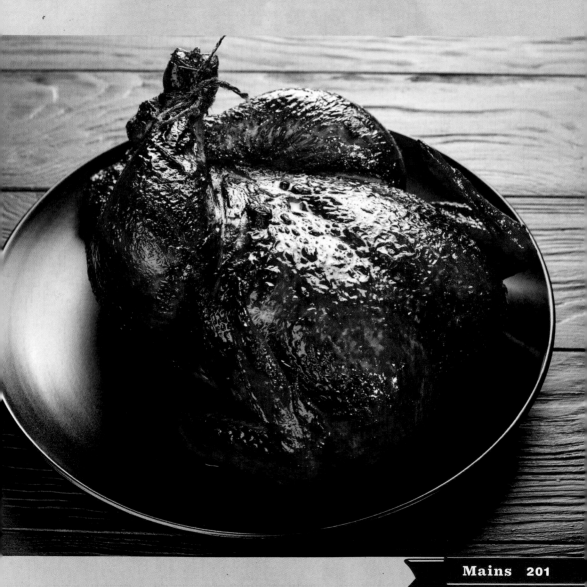

Slow Cooker Cornish Game Hens

YIELD: 6 SERVINGS • PREP TIME: 10 MINUTES • COOK TIME: 3½ TO 7½ HOURS
NUTRITIONAL INFO: CALORIES: 181 • FAT: 8G • NET CARBS: 3G • PROTEIN: 22G

The Cornish game hen is a young chicken that is not over 5 weeks of age, nor more than 2 lbs. It's the result of crossing the Cornish Game and White Plymouth Rock chicken breeds.

INGREDIENTS

2 tablespoons olive oil

1 small onion, minced

1 garlic clove, minced

2 small Cornish game hens, split in two, skin removed (approx. 20 oz.)

½ lbs. Swiss chard, washed, coarse stems removed, and leaves chopped in large pieces

½ lbs. escarole, washed, trimmed, and chopped in large pieces

½ cup chicken stock or broth

1 lb. baby spinach leaves

Salt and pepper, to taste

1 Heat oil in a small skillet over medium-high heat. Cook the onion and garlic for about 3 minutes, or until the onion is translucent. Scrape mixture into slow cooker.

2 Place Cornish hens on top of onion mixture, and top with Swiss chard, escarole, and stock.

3 Cover the slow cooker and cook on Low for 6 to 7 hours or on High for 3 to 4 hours, or until chicken is tender and cooked through.

4 Add the baby spinach and cook for another 20 to 30 minutes. Season with salt and pepper and serve.

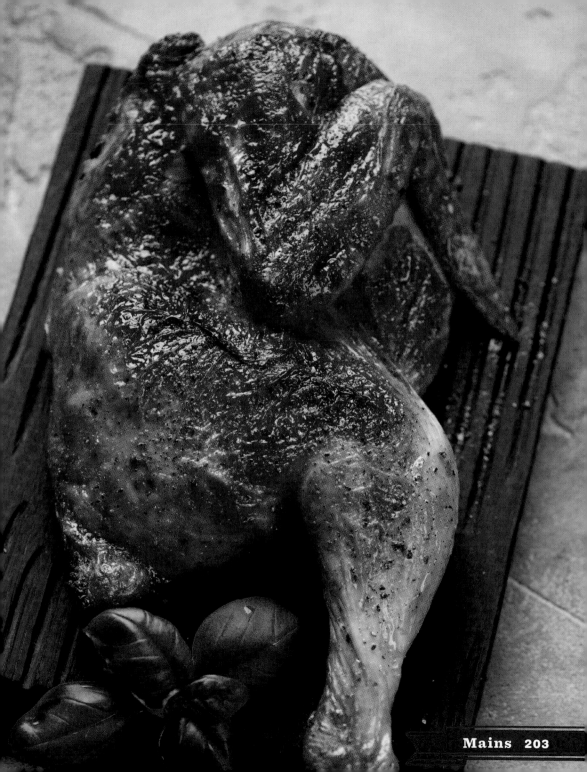

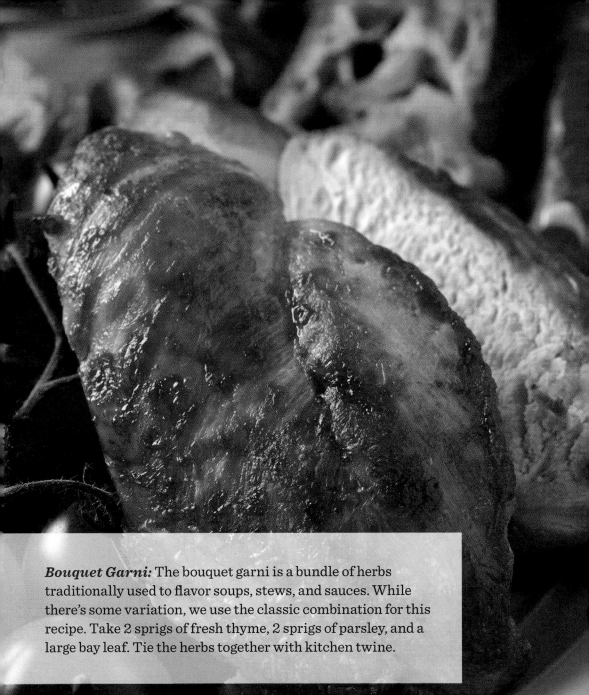

Bouquet Garni: The bouquet garni is a bundle of herbs traditionally used to flavor soups, stews, and sauces. While there's some variation, we use the classic combination for this recipe. Take 2 sprigs of fresh thyme, 2 sprigs of parsley, and a large bay leaf. Tie the herbs together with kitchen twine.

Slow Cooker Poached Chicken

YIELD: 6 SERVINGS • PREP TIME: 10 MINUTES • COOK TIME: 7 TO 10 HOURS
NUTRITIONAL INFO (FOR BREASTS): CALORIES: 96 • FAT: 14G • NET CARBS: 0G •
PROTEIN: 4G
NUTRITIONAL INFO (FOR COOKING LIQUID): CALORIES: 210 • FAT: 14G •
NET CARBS: 14G • PROTEIN: 4G

This dish is quite low in fat so it's best to serve the chicken shredded in a salad with some homemade mayonnaise or a tablespoon of oil. The left-over cooking liquid can work well in soups and stews.

1 Place chicken breasts in the slow cooker.

2 Heat oil in a skillet and add the onion and garlic. Cook until the onion is translucent, about 3 to 5 minutes. Transfer the onion mixture to the slow cooker. Cover the breasts with the chicken broth and water and squeeze the lemon over everything. Add the peppercorns and the bouquet garni.

3 Cover and cook on Low for 8 to 10 hours or on High for about 7 hours. Remove the bouquet garni after 4 hours. Remove the cooked chicken with a slotted spoon and allow to cool thoroughly. Put in a bowl covered with plastic wrap and serve cold.

INGREDIENTS

6 boneless, skinless chicken breasts (approx. 24 oz.)

1 tablespoon extra virgin olive oil

1 onion, chopped fine

2 garlic cloves, minced

2 cups chicken broth

2 cups water

½ lemon

1 teaspoon whole white peppercorns

1 bouquet garni (see sidebar)

Easy Turkey Breast

YIELD: 6 SERVINGS • PREP TIME: 5 MINUTES • COOK TIME: 6 TO 9 HOURS
NUTRITIONAL INFO: CALORIES: 512 • FAT: 15G • NET CARBS: 0G • PROTEIN: 91G

This recipe makes for turkey that can be used to top salads, rolled in lettuce leaves, or even eaten straight out of the fridge.

INGREDIENTS

4 lbs. boneless, skinless turkey breast

½ teaspoon salt

¼ teaspoon pepper

1 tablespoon fresh rosemary, chopped

1 tablespoon fresh parsley, chopped

½ cup chicken stock or broth

5 tablespoons melted butter

1 Place the turkey in the slow cooker. Sprinkle with salt and pepper, then add the herbs and stock.

2 Cover and cook on Low for 7 to 9 hours or on High for 4 to 6 hours, until the meat is cooked through. Pour melted butter over before serving.

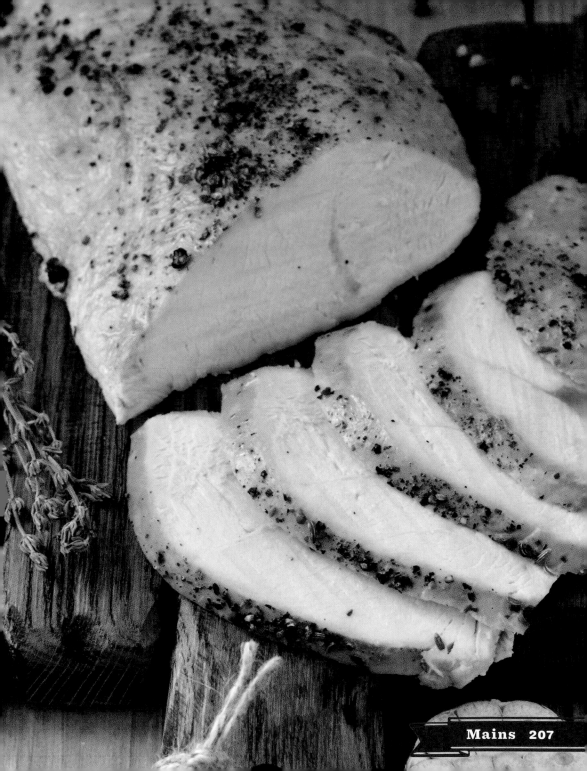

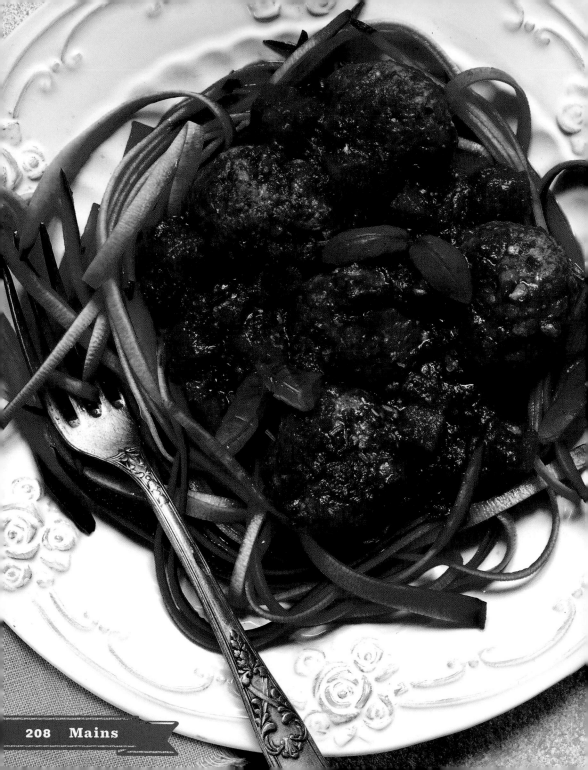

Slow Cooker Turkey Meatballs and Zucchini

YIELD: 6 SERVINGS • PREP TIME: 10 MINUTES • COOK TIME: 3 TO 6 HOURS
NUTRITIONAL INFO: CALORIES: 146 • FAT: 6G • NET CARBS: 5G • PROTEIN: 17G

You can substitute any other kind of ground meat in this recipe. You can also vary the spices to create different flavor profiles. Add some heavy cream or butter over each serving for more fat.

1 In a large bowl, combine the turkey, egg, onion, parsley, garlic, and a sprinkling of salt and pepper. Stir thoroughly.

2 Put the zucchini slices in the slow cooker. Form the turkey mixture into meatballs and put them on top of the zucchini. Pour the tomatoes over everything.

3 Cover and cook on Low for 4 to 6 hours or on High for 3 to 4 hours, until meatballs are cooked through and zucchini is tender. Season with additional salt and pepper, if desired.

INGREDIENTS

1 lb. ground turkey

1 egg

½ onion, minced

1 tablespoon fresh parsley, chopped fine

2 garlic cloves, pressed

Salt and pepper, to taste

2 large zucchini, sliced thin

14 oz. fresh tomatoes, pureed

Cajun-Blackened Tilapia

YIELD: 4 SERVINGS • PREP TIME: 15 MINUTES • COOK TIME: 6 MINUTES
NUTRITIONAL INFO: CALORIES: 378 • FAT: 4G • NET CARBS: 4G • PROTEIN: 21G

Tilapia is a wonderful fish for blackening, as it is a firm-fleshed fish that is fairly bland and benefits from seasoning. You can blacken many kinds of seafood, including catfish, tuna, grouper, halibut, trout, and even shrimp.

INGREDIENTS

For the Cajun Seasoning

1 tablespoon paprika

1 tablespoon onion powder

1 tablespoon garlic powder

2 tablespoons cayenne pepper

1 tablespoon white pepper

1 tablespoon ground black pepper

1 tablespoon dried thyme

1 tablespoon dried oregano

For the Tilapia

4 boneless tilapia fillets (approx. 4 oz. each)

1 stick butter, melted, plus 2 tablespoons butter, softened

1 lemon, cut into 4 wedges, for garnish

1 In a bowl, combine all the spices for your seasoning and set aside.

2 Heat the skillet over high heat for about 10 minutes until very hot. While the skillet heats, rinse the fillets and then pat dry with paper towels. Dip the fish fillets in the melted butter, covering both sides, and then press the blackened seasoning generously into both sides.

3 Put the fish in the skillet and cook for about 3 minutes a side, placing the softened butter on the tops while the bottoms cook. Serve with lemon.

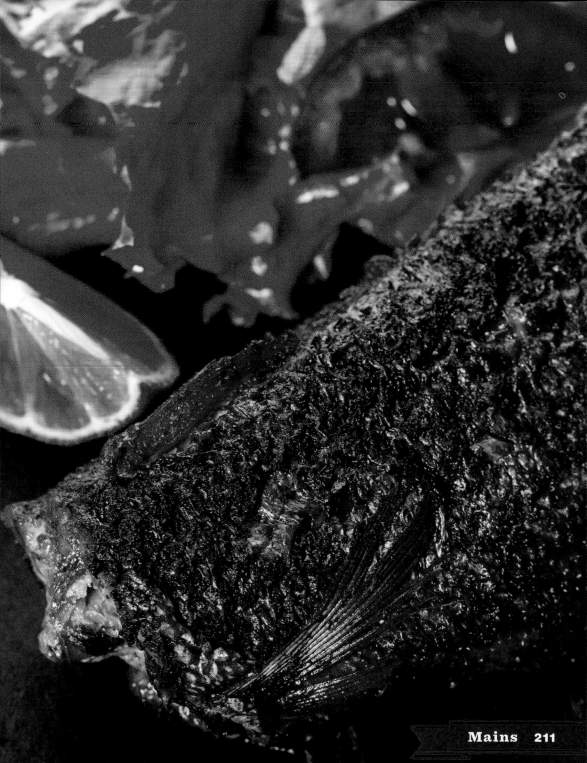

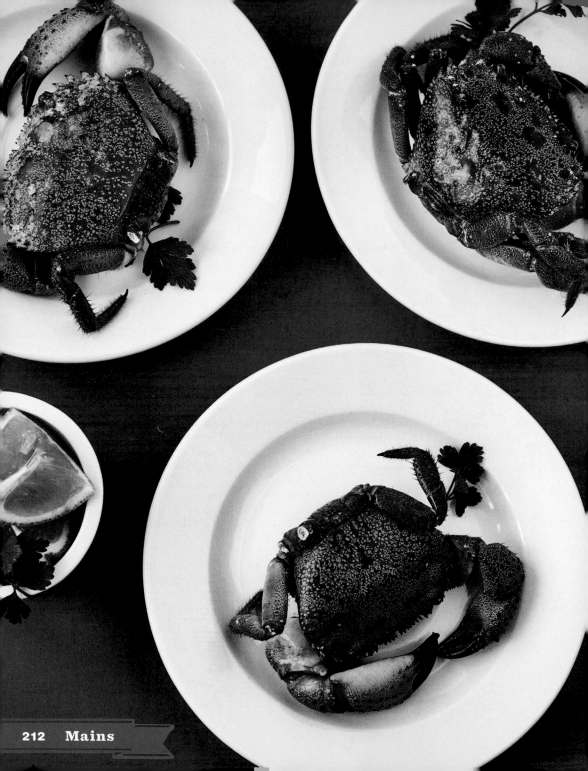

Chesapeake Blue Crabs

YIELD: 4 SERVINGS • PREP TIME: 5 MINUTES • COOK TIME: 3 HOURS
NUTRITIONAL INFO: CALORIES: 505 • FAT: 27G • NET CARBS: 0G • PROTEIN: 62G

It's worth the splurge to order Chesapeake blue crabs online. They arrive super-fresh and ready to cook and eat.

1 In a bowl, mix the water, vinegar, seasoning, and salt until well combined. Pour into the slow cooker. Cover and turn to High.

2 After 1 hour, add the crabs. Cover again and continue to cook on High for about 2 more hours, until the crabs have turned bright red and cooked through.

3 Divide the butter into bowls for dipping and serve alongside the crabs.

INGREDIENTS

2 cups water

½ cup distilled vinegar

¼ cup Old Bay Seasoning

1 tablespoon salt

3 lbs. blue crabs

½ cup unsalted butter, melted

Chili-Tomato Grilled Red Snapper

YIELD: 4 SERVINGS • PREP TIME: 10 MINUTES • COOK TIME: 10 MINUTES
NUTRITIONAL INFO (FOR GRILLED SNAPPER): CALORIES: 282 • FAT: 10G •
NET CARBS: 1G • PROTEIN: 45G
NUTRITIONAL INFO (FOR SAUCE): CALORIES: 93 • FAT: 7G • NET CARBS: 5G •
PROTEIN: 1G

The acidity of the tomatoes balances the slight sweetness from the garlic to create a dish you won't believe is keto-friendly.

INGREDIENTS

For the Snapper

4 red snapper fillets, skin-on (about 1½ to 2 inches thick)

2 tablespoons olive oil

2 teaspoons red pepper flakes (optional)

Salt and pepper, to taste

For the Chili-Tomato Sauce

2 chili peppers of your choice

2 tablespoons olive oil

1 small shallot, finely chopped

2 garlic cloves, minced

2 large tomatoes, crushed

¼ cup fresh cilantro, finely chopped

1 tablespoon flat-leaf parsley, finely chopped

2 tablespoons fresh chives, finely chopped

Salt and pepper, to taste

1 Rub the snapper fillets with oil and then season with the red pepper flakes (if desired), salt, and pepper. Let stand at room temperature while preparing the grill and sauce.

2 A half hour before cooking, place a cast-iron skillet on your gas or charcoal grill and prepare to medium heat. Leave the grill covered while heating, as it will add a faint smoky flavor to the skillet.

3 When the grill is ready, at about 400°F with the coals lightly covered with ash, add the chili peppers and cook until they are charred and wrinkled. Remove from pan and transfer to a small cutting board. Let cool and then stem the chilies. Finely chop and set aside.

4 Add the oil to the cast-iron skillet. Once hot, add the shallot and garlic cloves and cook until the shallot is translucent and the garlic is golden, about 2 minutes. Add the finely chopped chilies into the pan and sear for 1 minute. Mix in the tomatoes and cook until they have broken down. Stir in the cilantro, parsley, and chives and sear for a few more minutes. Season with salt and pepper and transfer to a bowl. While the sauce is still hot, mash with a fork and cover with aluminum foil.

5 Place the seasoned snapper fillets on the grill directly over the heat source. Cover the grill and cook each side for about 3 minutes. When finished, the fillets should be opaque in the center and should easily tear when pierced with a fork. Transfer to a carving board and peel back the skin. Let rest 5 to 10 minutes, and then serve on beds of chili-tomato sauce.

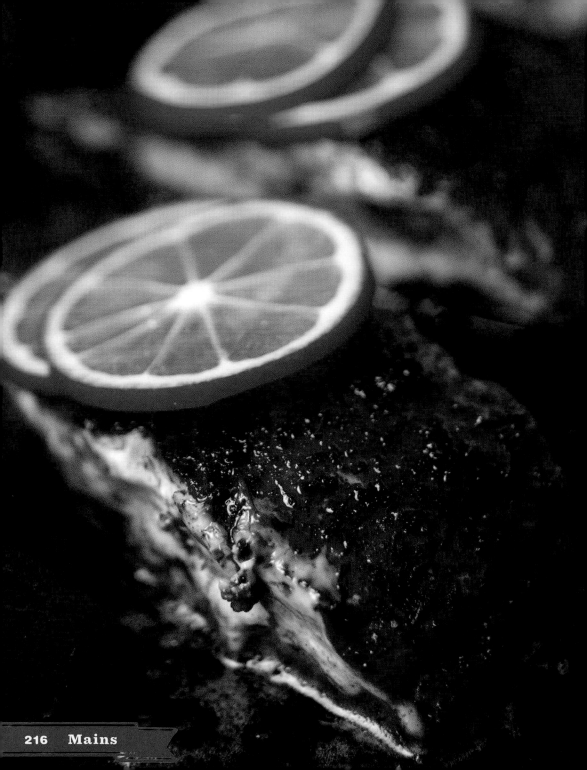

Easy Skillet Salmon

YIELD: 4 SERVINGS • PREP TIME: 5 MINUTES • COOK TIME: 5 MINUTES
NUTRITIONAL INFO: CALORIES: 521 • FAT: 31G • NET CARBS: 1G • PROTEIN: 57G

There are two different cuts of salmon: steaks and fillets. The steaks are cut from the meat around the backbone, and they contain bone in the middle. Fillets are cut from the flesh that extends from the head to the tail of the fish. For this recipe, use fillets. You can also toss some vegetables in the oil that remains in the pan after cooking for a delicious side.

1 Rinse the fillets with cold water to ensure that any scales or bones are removed. Dry them with paper towels. Rub some of the butter on both sides of the fillets, squeeze lemon over them, and season with salt and pepper.

2 Heat the skillet over medium-high heat and add the oil and unused butter. Add the fillets, flesh side down. Cook on one side for about 3 minutes, then flip them and cook for 2 minutes on the other side.

3 Remove the pan from the heat and let the fish rest in it for a minute before serving. The skin should peel right off. Pour the oils from the pan over the fish before serving.

INGREDIENTS

8 salmon fillets (approx. 4 oz. each)

2 tablespoons unsalted butter, cut in pieces, softened

1 lemon

Salt and pepper, to taste

1 tablespoon extra virgin olive oil

Grilled Tuna Steaks with Dill Aioli

YIELD: 4 SERVINGS • PREP TIME: 30 MINUTES • COOK TIME: ABOUT 6 MINUTES
NUTRITIONAL INFO: CALORIES: 547 • FAT: 50G • NET CARBS: 1G • PROTEIN: 26G

Seared tuna steaks are always a treat on a warm summer evening. You have the option of serving these steaks chilled or right off the grill. The dill aioli is perfect when served slightly chilled.

INGREDIENTS

For the Tuna Steaks

4 fresh tuna steaks (approx. 2 inches thick)

2 tablespoon extra virgin olive oil, plus a little extra for the grill

Salt and pepper, to taste

For the Dill Aioli

10 sprigs dill, finely chopped

10 sprigs parsley, finely chopped

Juice of ¼ small lemon

1 garlic clove, minced

¾ cup extra virgin olive oil, plus more for grill

Salt, to taste

1 Rub the tuna steaks with a little extra virgin olive oil and then season with salt and pepper. Let rest at room temperature while you prepare the grill and dill aioli.

2 Prepare your gas or charcoal grill to high heat.

3 While waiting for the grill, combine the dill, parsley, lemon juice, and garlic clove into a small bowl and whisk together. While whisking, slowly incorporate the oil and season with salt. Set aside or chill in the refrigerator. If you want a lighter aioli, combine the initial ingredients in a blender and then slowly add the oil.

4 When the grill is ready, at about 450°F to 500°F with the coals lightly covered with ash, brush the grate with a little oil. Tuna steaks should always be cooked between rare and medium-rare; anything more will be tough and dry. To accomplish a perfect searing, place the tuna steaks directly over the hot part of the coals and sear for about 2 minutes per side. The tuna should be raw in the middle (cook 2½ to 3 minutes per side for medium-rare).

5 Transfer the tuna steaks to a large carving board and let rest for 5 to 10 minutes. Slice against the grain, season with salt, and serve with dill aioli.

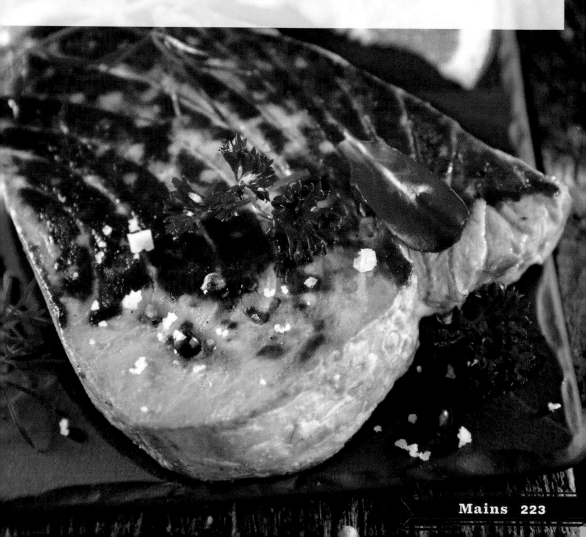

Pan-Seared Salmon in Bell Pepper Sauce

YIELD: 3 SERVINGS • PREP TIME: 15 MINUTES • COOK TIME: ABOUT 5 MINUTES
NUTRITIONAL INFO (FOR SAUCE): CALORIES: 130 • FAT: 12G • NET CARBS: 4G •
PROTEIN: 1G

These delicious, crispy salmon fillets with a creamy bell pepper sauce go incredibly well with a side of sautéed spinach.

INGREDIENTS

3 salmon fillets (approx. 5¼ oz. each)

1 teaspoon Old Bay Seasoning

1 tablespoon olive oil

1 tablespoon butter

2½ teaspoons garlic, chopped

¼ cup red bell peppers, diced

¼ cup yellow bell peppers, diced

¼ chicken bouillon cube

½ cup water, as needed

3¼ cups heavy whipping cream

1 teaspoon parsley, chopped

1 Start by prepping the salmon fillets. Score the skin with a sharp knife and then season generously with Old Bay. Alternatively, use salt, pepper, and any other spices of choice.

2 Heat the olive oil in a frying pan and place the salmon skin side down and cook for 2 minutes, until the skin is crispy. Flip over and cook for one more minute, and then on each side for about 30 seconds. When done, remove from the pan.

3 In the same skillet, heat the butter, add in the garlic and bell peppers, and sauté.

4 Season with the bouillon cube and add water as required to deglaze the pan. Cook until the liquid has reduced by half. Once you reach a gentle simmer, add cream and give it all a good mix.

5 Turn off the heat and finish with the freshly chopped parsley.

6 Plate the salmon and spoon a serving of sauce over each fillet.

NOTE: THE MACROS ARE JUST FOR THE SAUCE, SO MAKE SURE TO INPUT THE MACROS FOR THE SALMON SEPARATELY BASED ON THE WEIGHT OF THE FILLET. 3½ OZ. OF RAW ATLANTIC SALMON HAS 208 CALORIES, 13G OF FAT, 0G OF CARBS, AND 20G OF PROTEIN.

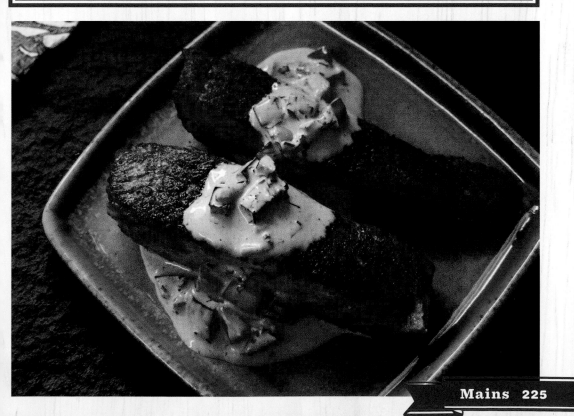

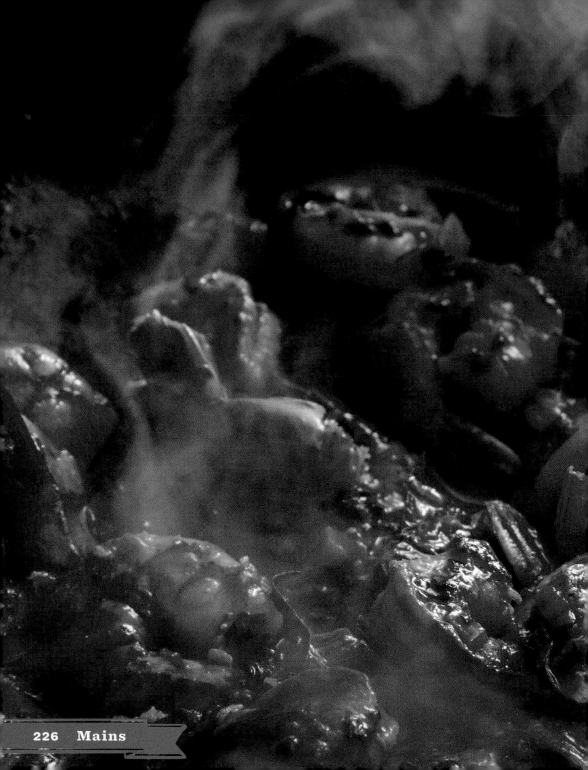

Shrimp Scampi

YIELD: 4 SERVINGS • PREP TIME: 5 MINUTES • COOK TIME: 2 TO 4 HOURS
NUTRITIONAL INFO: CALORIES: 356 • FAT: 16G • NET CARBS: 3G • PROTEIN: 48G

Make a meal out of this dish by serving the shrimp and sauce over spaghetti squash.

1 Heat the oil and butter in a skillet and add the garlic, stirring until it sizzles. Add the tomatoes, red pepper flakes, oregano, salt, and pepper. Stir to combine and cook for about 3 minutes. Add in the water and bring to a boil.

2 Transfer sauce to the slow cooker. Place the shrimp on the sauce. Cover and cook on Low for 4 hours or on High for about 2 hours, until the shrimp are cooked through.

3 Serve straight out of the slow cooker with long forks or toothpicks.

INGREDIENTS

2 tablespoons extra virgin olive oil

2 tablespoons butter

4 garlic cloves, minced

2 tomatoes, chopped

1 tablespoon red pepper flakes

1 teaspoon oregano

Salt and pepper, to taste

2 cups water

2 lbs. medium-sized raw shrimp, shells removed

Slow Cooker Bluefish with Lemon and Tarragon

YIELD: 4 SERVINGS • PREP TIME: 10 MINUTES • COOK TIME: 1 TO 4 HOURS
NUTRITIONAL INFO: CALORIES: 545 • FAT: 26G • NET CARBS: 4G • PROTEIN: 69G

This simply prepared fish is also delicious chilled and served in lettuce wraps. Just garnish with chopped cucumbers, cherry tomatoes, and a thin slice of avocado.

INGREDIENTS

3 lbs. bluefish fillets

2 tablespoons fresh tarragon, chopped

2 lemons

1 medium onion, thinly sliced

4 tablespoons butter

Salt and pepper, to taste

1 Make sure the fillets are free of bones. Put them skin side down into the slow cooker.

2 Sprinkle the tarragon over the fish, then squeeze the lemons over them. Remove any seeds. Thinly slice one of the squeezed lemons and place the slices on the fish. Finally, top with the onion slices and butter and season with salt and pepper.

3 Cook on Low for 3 to 4 hours or on High for 1 to 2 hours, until fish is cooked through and very flaky.

Crab-Stuffed Salmon Fillets

YIELD: 6 SERVINGS • PREP TIME: 15 MINUTES • COOK TIME: 4 TO 5 HOURS
NUTRITIONAL INFO: CALORIES: 415 • FAT: 23G • NET CARBS: 2G • PROTEIN: 51G

Spinach makes an excellent accompaniment to stuffed salmon fillets. Steam baby spinach leaves and make a pile of them in the center of a dinner plate. Place the stuffed salmon on top and serve with a wedge of lemon on the side.

INGREDIENTS

8 oz. cooked crabmeat (fresh or imitation), flaked

¼ cup celery, minced

2 garlic cloves, minced

¼ cup red bell pepper, minced

1 teaspoon fresh parsley, chopped fine

¼ teaspoon salt

½ teaspoon freshly ground pepper

1 teaspoon fresh lemon juice

1 egg

¼ cup unsalted butter, melted

5 salmon fillets (approx. 6 oz. each)

1 Make the crabmeat stuffing by combining the crabmeat, celery, garlic, red pepper, parsley, salt, pepper, lemon juice, egg, and melted butter in a bowl. Stir well to combine.

2 Make a slit in the side of the salmon fillets and evenly divide the stuffing between the fillets. Gently transfer each stuffed fillet to the slow cooker.

3 Cover and cook on Low for 4 to 5 hours, until the fish is cooked through.

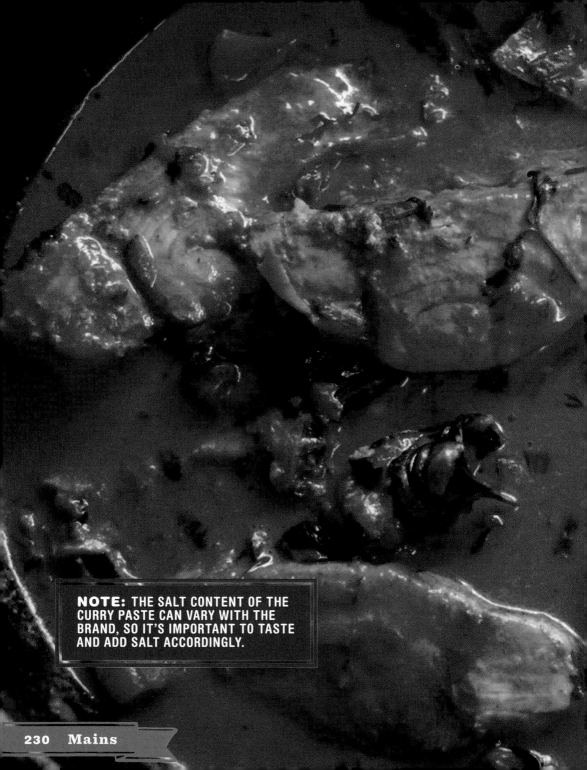

NOTE: THE SALT CONTENT OF THE CURRY PASTE CAN VARY WITH THE BRAND, SO IT'S IMPORTANT TO TASTE AND ADD SALT ACCORDINGLY.

Yellow Thai Fish Curry

YIELD: 3 SERVINGS • PREP TIME: 5 MINUTES • COOK TIME: ABOUT 5 MINUTES
NUTRITIONAL INFO: CALORIES: 371 • FAT: 26G • NET CARBS: 3G • PROTEIN: 32G

A mild white fish like cod or hake is an ideal complement to this spicy, yellow Thai curry.

1 Heat the coconut oil in a wok and then fry the curry paste for a minute until fragrant.

2 Pour in about half of the coconut milk to create the curry base, and then add the grated zucchini and cook for a minute.

3 Next, then add the boy choy and the rest of the coconut milk and cook for 3 to 4 minutes before placing the fish in the curry.

4 Cook the fish until it is cooked through, check the seasoning, garnish with cilantro, and serve.

INGREDIENTS

1 tablespoon coconut oil

2 tablespoons Thai yellow curry paste

1 cup coconut milk

1¼ cups zucchini, grated

1 cup bok choy

15¾ oz. Kingfish (or any white fish of choice)

Salt, as needed

Cilantro, for garnish

Classic Ratatouille

YIELD: 4 TO 6 SERVINGS • PREP TIME: 45 MINUTES
COOK TIME: 40 TO 45 MINUTES
NUTRITIONAL INFO: CALORIES: 133 • FAT: 10G • NET CARBS: 6G • PROTEIN: 3G

To add more protein to this dish, sear top round beef cut into bite-sized pieces brushed with extra virgin olive oil until they become golden brown. Add this to the saucepan with the grilled vegetables.

INGREDIENTS

1 medium eggplant

1 medium summer squash

1 medium zucchini

1 medium onion

Salt and pepper, to taste

3 tablespoons olive oil

2 garlic cloves, minced

1 (14 oz.) can stewed tomatoes

¼ cup parsley, minced

Pinch of dried basil

Pinch of oregano

¼ cup basil leaves

1 Prepare vegetables by cutting eggplant into ½-inch pieces, the summer squash and zucchini in half lengthwise, and onion into quarters. Wash the eggplant pieces and sprinkle with salt. Let sit for 30 minutes.

2 In a large bowl, pour 2 tablespoons of oil. Add eggplant, squash, zucchini, and onion to the bowl and toss to coat. Preheat grill to medium-high heat. Place eggplant, squash, and zucchini directly on the grill. Skewer the onion before placing on the grill. Grill vegetables until they are lightly charred: about 10 to 12 minutes for the onion, and 4 to 5 minutes per side for the eggplant, squash, and zucchini. Remove from heat and let cool.

3 Cut the squash and zucchini into slivers. Add 1 tablespoon of oil to a large saucepan and then cook garlic over low heat until the garlic is golden, about 2 minutes. Stir in the grilled vegetables, stewed tomatoes, parsley, dried basil, oregano, salt, and pepper. Cook for about 30 minutes. Stir in the basil leaves and then serve.

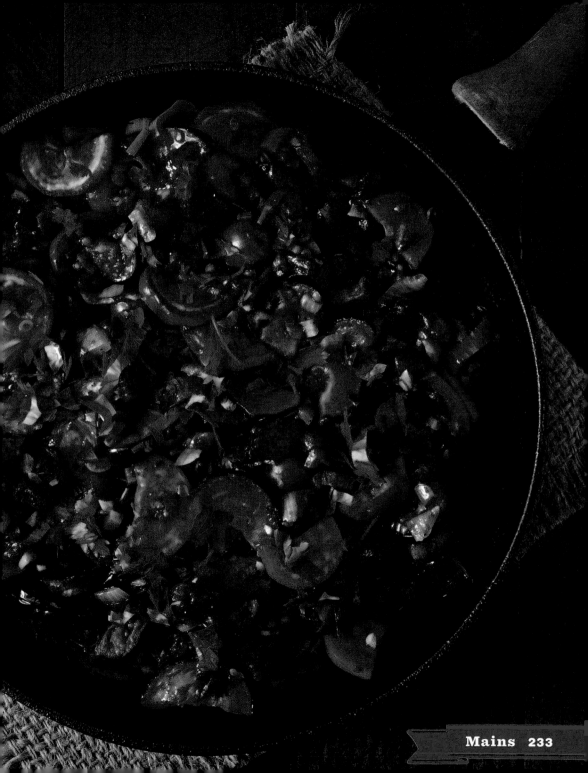

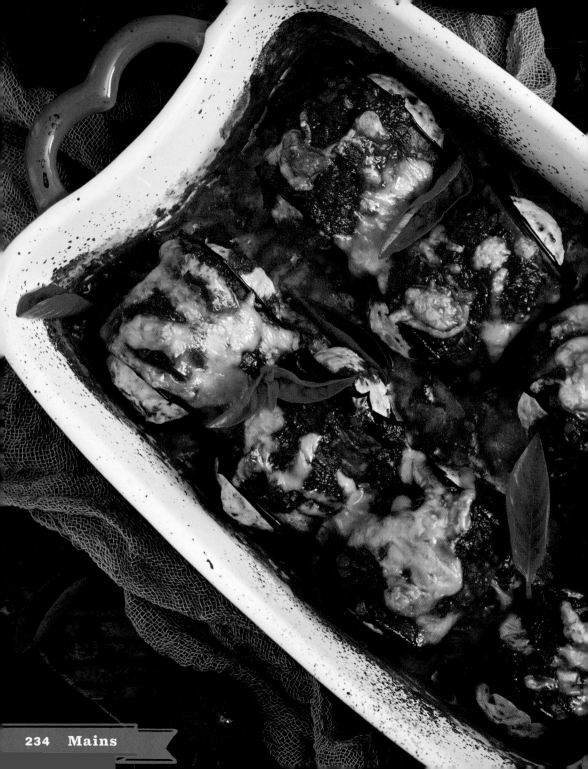

Eggplant Rollatini

YIELD: 4 SERVINGS • PREP TIME: 30 MINUTES • COOK TIME: 12 MINUTES
NUTRITIONAL INFO: CALORIES: 508 • FAT: 42G • NET CARBS: 15G • PROTEIN: 15G

Bacon bits make a great addition to this cheesy spread.

1 Slice eggplant lengthwise to yield 12 slices. Place the slices in a colander and salt them.

2 After letting the slices drain for 20 minutes, dry and coat them in oil, salt, and pepper.

3 Preheat grill to medium heat. Grill the slices for 10 minutes, flipping them over halfway through. Cook your slices until grill marks appear and they become slightly tender. Remove from heat and allow them to cool.

4 In a medium-sized bowl, mix together the ricotta, lemon zest, basil, nutmeg, and as much Parmesan as you want.

5 Once everything is properly mixed, lay out your eggplant slices. Add a few tablespoons of the mixture to the end closest to you. Roll up the eggplant and secure with a toothpick.

6 Grill the eggplant for about 2 more minutes, remove from heat, and serve.

TOOLS

Handful of toothpicks

INGREDIENTS

3 medium-sized eggplants

½ cup extra virgin olive oil

Salt and pepper, to taste

1½ cups ricotta

Zest of ½ lemon

1 tablespoon basil, chopped

pinch of nutmeg, freshly grated

Parmesan cheese, to taste

Goat Cheese-Stuffed Zucchini

YIELD: 4 SERVINGS • PREP TIME: 10 MINUTES • COOK TIME: 10 MINUTES
NUTRITIONAL INFO: CALORIES: 353 • FAT: 24G • NET CARBS: 9G • PROTEIN: 23G

For more protein, add chopped up ham to the zucchini log when you add the goat cheese. Use a homemade marinara sauce for less carbs and add a tablespoon of butter before serving for more fat.

INGREDIENTS

4 medium-sized zucchini

Salt and pepper, to taste

3 cups goat cheese

2 cups marinara sauce

1 Preheat the grill to high heat. Slice your zucchini in half lengthwise. Hollow out the zucchini by removing seeds to create a trough. Season the halves with salt and pepper.

2 Evenly spread the goat cheese in the troughs of each zucchini, using as little or as much as you'd like. Repeat the process with the marinara sauce.

3 Grill the logs until the cheese becomes soft and the marinara is bubbling slightly. This should take about 10 minutes. Remove from heat and serve.

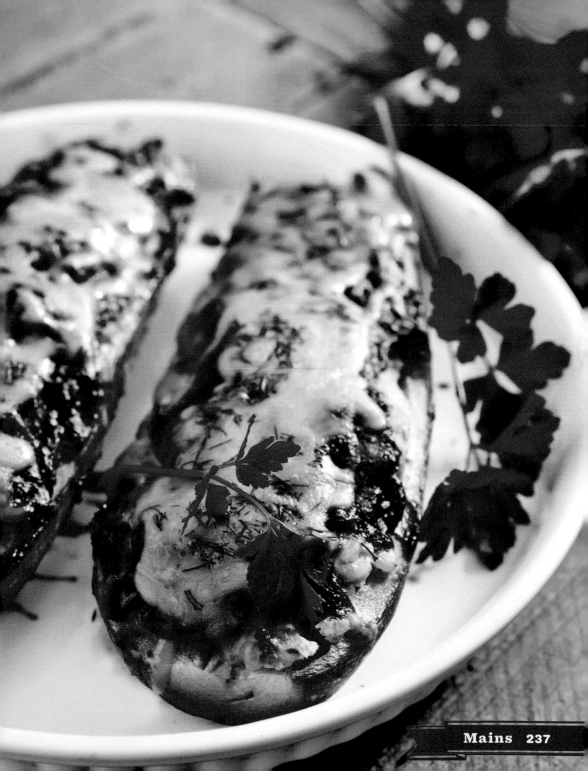

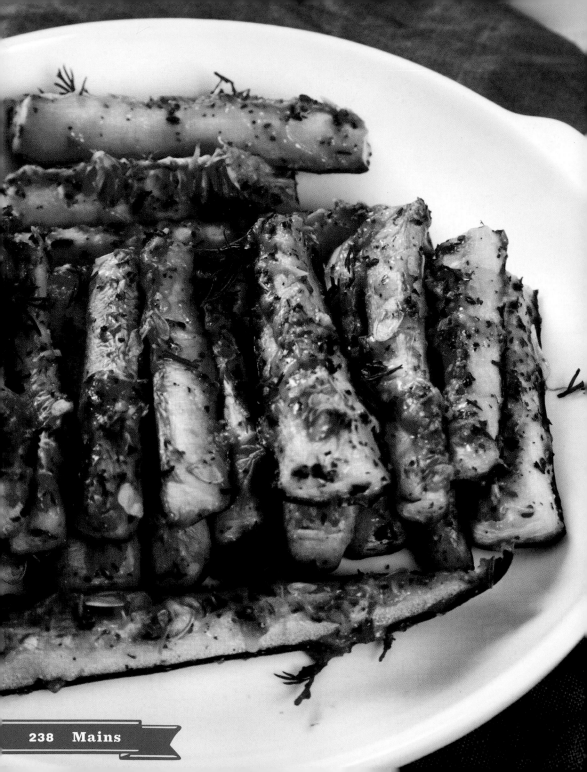

Grilled Zucchini Parmesan

YIELD: 4 SERVINGS • PREP TIME: 10 MINUTES • COOK TIME: ABOUT 8 MINUTES
NUTRITIONAL INFO: CALORIES: 347 • FAT: 27G • NET CARBS: 5G • PROTEIN: 21G

You can always add chicken to this recipe or use it as a replacement for the zucchini. Coat 1 pound of skinless, boneless chicken in the same way you'd coat the zucchini and grill for 5 to 6 minutes per side, or until it is completely cooked through. Top with mozzarella cheese and cook until the cheese melts.

1 Preheat grill to medium-high heat. Oil the grill to prevent sticking. Cut each zucchini lengthwise into four pieces. In a small bowl, mix together the oil, butter, garlic, and parsley. Add salt to the mixture, to taste. Use this mixture to coat the zucchini slices.

2 Place the zucchini slices on the hot grates and grill until the slices are tender. This should take about 8 minutes. Sprinkle one side of the zucchini with Parmesan cheese. Remove from heat and serve.

INGREDIENTS

2 tablespoons olive oil, plus more for grill

3 medium zucchini

2 tablespoons butter, softened

2 garlic cloves, minced

1 tablespoon parsley, chopped

Salt, to taste

½ cup Parmesan cheese, grated

Indian-Chinese Hakka Noodles

YIELD: 3 SERVINGS • PREP TIME: 15 MINUTES
COOK TIME: ABOUT 5 MINUTES
NUTRITIONAL INFO (PER SERVING): CALORIES: 269 • FAT: 9G •
NET CARBS: 5G • PROTEIN: 37G

Meat noodles make this popular Indian-Chinese stir fry a keto staple.

INGREDIENTS

1 tablespoon olive oil

2 garlic cloves, chopped

1 spring onion, chopped, white and green sections separated

½ cup green bell pepper, sliced

1½ cups mushrooms, sliced

¼ cup cabbage, sliced

Salt and pepper, to taste

7 oz. cooked Chicken Noodles (see page 85)

1 teaspoon black vinegar

1 teaspoon soy sauce

1 teaspoon Sriracha

1 Heat up the oil in a wok and fry the garlic and spring onion whites. Once the garlic starts to brown, add in all the vegetables and sauté them, seasoning with salt and pepper.

2 Once the vegetables have softened, add the Chicken Noodles and warm through.

3 Add the vinegar, soy sauce, and Sriracha and mix well.

4 Garnish with spring onion greens and serve.

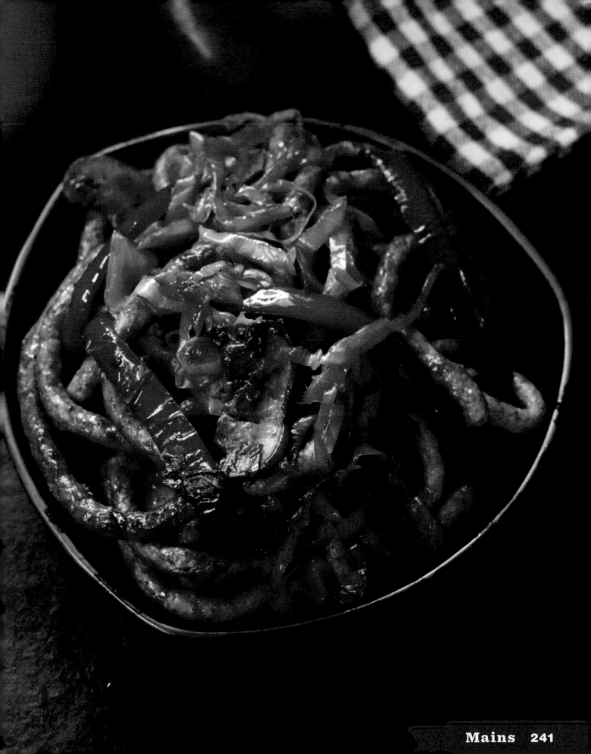

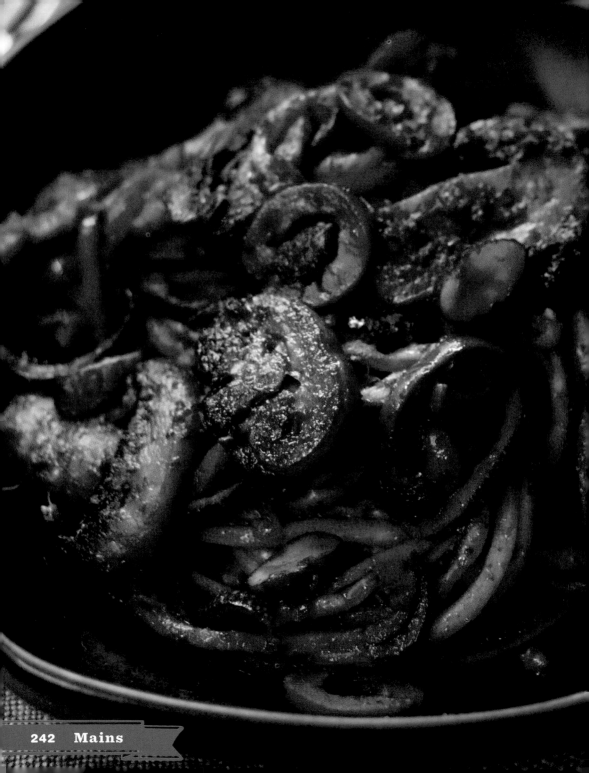

Pesto Zoodles with Mushrooms and Olives

YIELD: 1 SERVING • PREP TIME: 10 MINUTES • COOK TIME: ABOUT 5 MINUTES
NUTRITIONAL INFO: CALORIES: 378 • FAT: 36G • NET CARBS: 8G • PROTEIN: 5G

This delicious low-carb "spaghetti" is a great vegetarian keto meal.

1 Spiralize the zucchini to make the spaghetti or use a peeler to make linguini-like strips.

2 Heat oil in a frying pan and fry the mushrooms, seasoning with salt and pepper. Then, add the olives, cooking until both they and the mushrooms begin to brown.

3 Add the zucchini and cook for 1 minute, then add the pesto and mix well.

4 Cook for another minute and serve.

INGREDIENTS

1 medium zucchini

6 white mushrooms, sliced

Salt and pepper, to taste

6 almond-stuffed olives, sliced

1 tablespoon olive oil

1½ tablespoons Basil Pesto (see page 105)

Vegetarian Thai Curry

YIELD: 5 SERVINGS • PREP TIME: 15 MINUTES • COOK TIME: 10 MINUTES
NUTRITIONAL INFO: CALORIES: 298 • FAT: 28G • NET CARBS: 6G • PROTEIN: 5G

This veggie-rich, Thai-style coconut curry makes for a hearty, meat-free meal.

INGREDIENTS

2½ cups coconut milk, plus more as needed

1 lemongrass stalk

1-inch piece of ginger, sliced

4 kaffir lime leaves, torn up

3¾ tablespoons Thai green curry paste

1 small zucchini, chopped

½ cup broccoli, chopped

1½ cups button mushrooms, sliced

2 or 3 small Thai eggplants

Salt, to taste

Stevia, to taste

Thai basil leaves, to taste

Riced Cauliflower (see page 81), for serving

1 Heat a wok over medium heat and add about ½ cup of coconut milk. When bubbles start to form at the edge of the liquid, bruise the lemongrass stalk and add it to the wok, along with the ginger and 2 kaffir lime leaves.

2 Add the green curry paste and stir it all together until it becomes fragrant. When the oil starts to separate from the paste, add the vegetables and stir until everything is coated with the paste.

3 Add the rest of the coconut milk. If curry is too thick, add additional coconut milk to thin the mixture.

4 Add salt to taste and a few drops of stevia to impart the mildest sweetness. Give it all a stir, then cover and let the veggies cook.

5 When the veggies are almost tender, add the remaining kaffir lime leaves to refresh the taste.

6 Once veggies are cooked to desired consistency, remove pan from heat and stir in a handful of Thai basil leaves.

7 Serve with Riced Cauliflower.

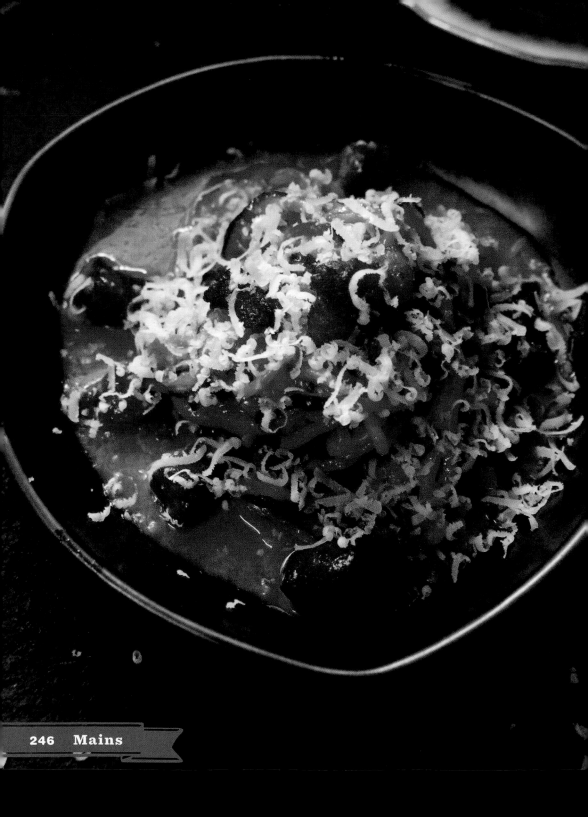

Zucchini Carbonara

YIELD: 2 SERVINGS • PREP TIME: 10 MINUTES • COOK TIME: 5 MINUTES
NUTRITIONAL INFO: CALORIES: 601 • FAT: 54G • NET CARBS: 2G • PROTEIN: 24G

This filling zucchini noodle dish will make you forget you're not eating pasta.

1 Mix together the egg, egg yolk, Parmesan, and black pepper.

2 Spiralize the zucchini to make the spaghetti or use a peeler to make linguini-like strips.

3 Fry the bacon, starting out in a cold pan to render out the fat. Once the fat has rendered and the bacon is crisp, remove excess grease, if any.

4 Add the zucchini, season with salt, and cook until tender.

5 Take the pan off the heat, pour in the egg mixture, and fold until the zucchini is well coated.

6 Garnish with freshly grated Parmesan and serve.

INGREDIENTS

1 egg, plus 1 yolk

3¾ tablespoons Parmesan cheese, grated, plus more for garnish

Black pepper and salt, to taste

2 medium zucchini

7 oz. smoked bacon, diced

Cauliflower Pizza Dough

YIELD: 4 SERVINGS • PREP TIME: 15 MINUTES TO 8 HOURS
COOK TIME: 30 MINUTES
NUTRITIONAL INFO: CALORIES: 326 • FAT: 21G • NET CARBS: 4G • PROTEIN: 29G

This pizza dough is also perfect for anyone following another low-carb diet. Just make sure the cauliflower is completely dry before processing it.

INGREDIENTS

12 oz. bag frozen cauliflower

¼ cup Parmesan cheese, grated

2 cups mozzarella, shredded

3 teaspoons oregano

1 teaspoon basil

½ teaspoon salt

1 garlic clove, minced

2 eggs, lightly beaten

1 Steam the cauliflower according to the directions on the package. Cook the cauliflower ahead of time and let it dry overnight on a sheet pan in the refrigerator, or let it cool and pat dry. This will help get all of the water out and keep the crust as crisp as possible.

2 Pulse the completely dry cauliflower in a food processor and add it to a large bowl.

3 Add the Parmesan, mozzarella, oregano, basil, salt, garlic, and eggs. Mix well and transfer mixture to a baking sheet.

4 Spread it into a large circle and bake for 20 minutes. After adding your pizza toppings, cook for another 10 minutes on the grill over medium heat.

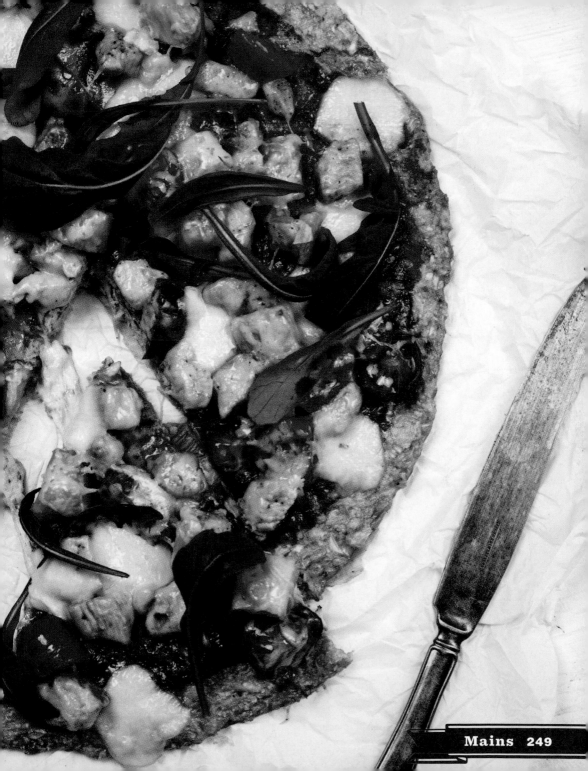

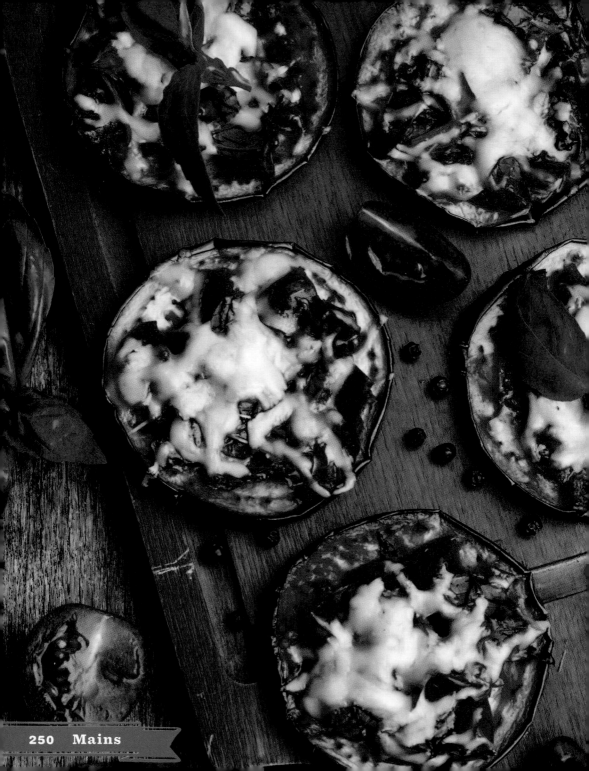

Grilled Eggplant Pizzas

YIELD: 4 SERVINGS • PREP TIME: 1 HOUR 15 MINUTES
COOK TIME: ABOUT 5 MINUTES
NUTRITIONAL INFO: CALORIES: 295 • FAT: 23G • NET CARBS: 11G • PROTEIN: 7G

To add some protein, grill up a few slices of prosciutto and tear them, spreading evenly across the eggplant pizza.

INGREDIENTS

- 3 lbs. eggplant
- 3 tablespoons salt
- ⅓ cup extra virgin olive oil
- Pepper, to taste
- 1 cup low-carb pizza sauce
- ½ cup mozzarella cheese
- Parmesan cheese

1 Cut your eggplant into ½-inch slices, sprinkling salt on both sides of every slice. Place the slices in a colander over your sink or in a bowl. Let this stand for 1 hour to drain. Rinse the slices under cold water, place on several layers of paper towels, and press the water out.

2 Preheat the grill to medium-high heat. Brush both sides of the slices with oil and sprinkle with pepper. Place your slices on the grill and cook one side until it is slightly browned, about 5 to 6 minutes.

3 Once that first side has cooked, flip the slice over and remove from heat. Distribute sauce and mozzarella over the grilled side of the slice.

4 Place eggplant back on the grill to cook the other side and melt the cheese. Remove from grill, top with Parmesan cheese, and serve.

Grilled Portobello Pizzas

YIELD: 4 SERVINGS • PREP TIME: 1 HOUR 10 MINUTES • COOK TIME: 10 MINUTES
NUTRITIONAL INFO: CALORIES: 399 • FAT: 32G • NET CARBS: 7G • PROTEIN: 24G

Top the mushrooms with ½ cup of pepperoni slices to enhance the savory flavor.

INGREDIENTS

¼ cup extra virgin olive oil

4 garlic cloves, minced

2 tablespoons balsamic vinegar

8 large portobello mushroom caps

1 cup tomato sauce

2 cups mozzarella cheese, grated

1 cup Parmesan cheese, grated

Fresh basil leaves, for garnish

1 In a large resealable bag, mix together the oil, garlic, and balsamic vinegar. Once you've combined the mixture, place the mushroom caps in the bag and let them marinate for 1 hour.

2 After the caps have marinated, fill them with about ¼ cup of tomato sauce and top with freshly grated mozzarella, then with Parmesan.

3 Preheat grill to medium heat and place the caps on the grill for about 10 minutes, or until cheese melts. Remove from heat, top with torn basil leaves, and serve.

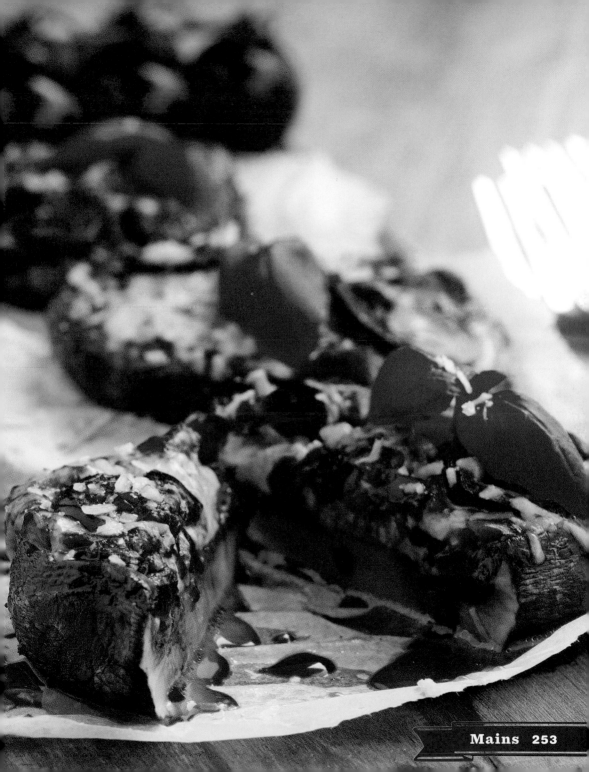

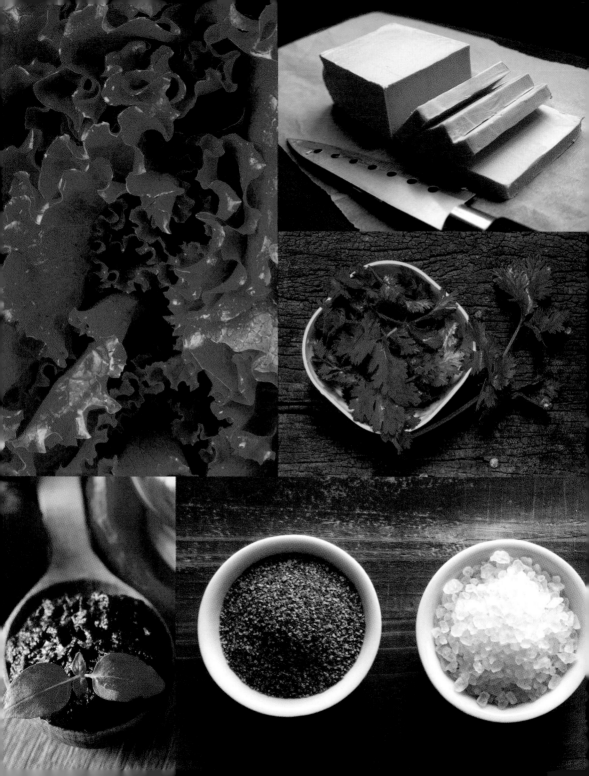

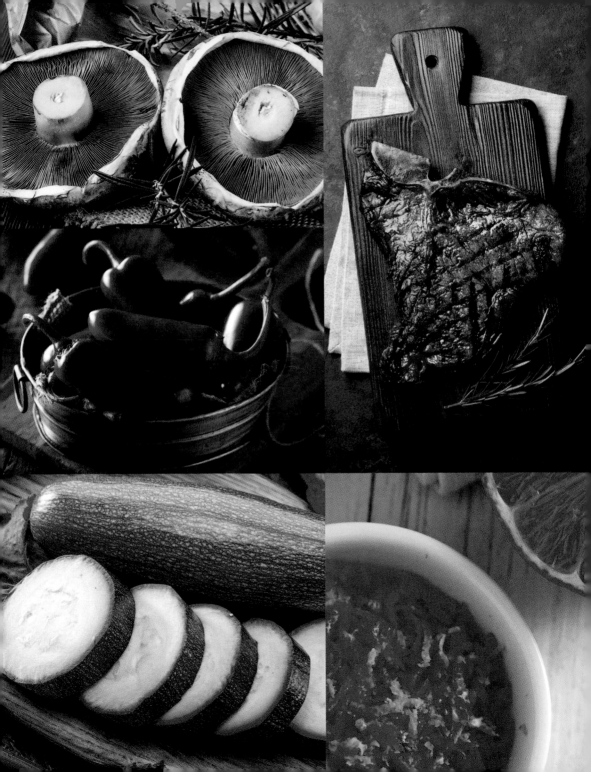

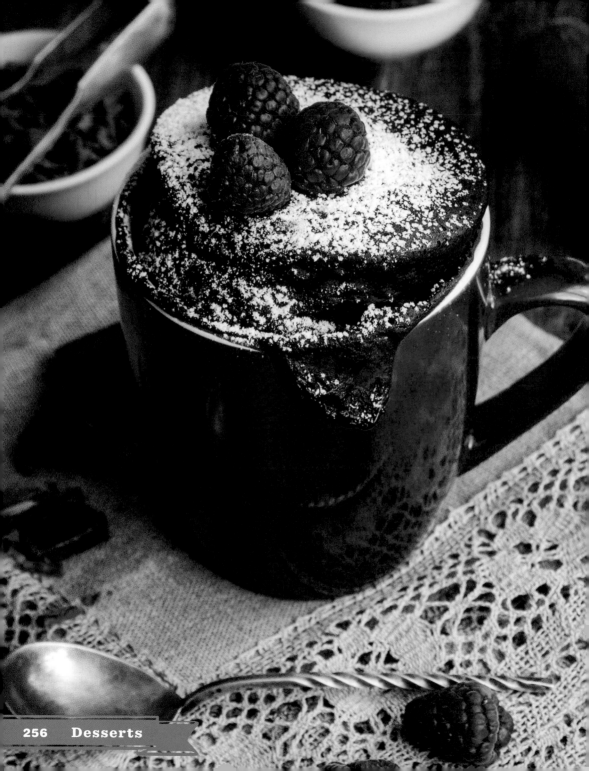

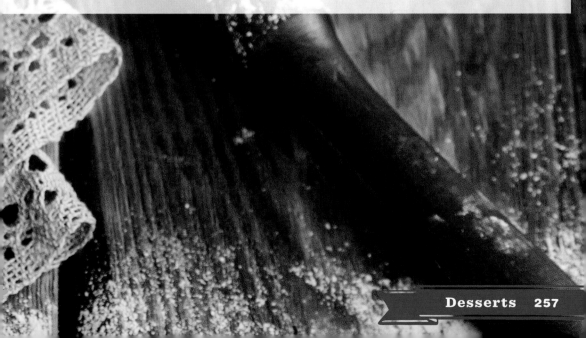

Desserts

While sugar should be avoided when on keto, that doesn't mean you have to give up sweet after-dinner indulgences. Heavy cream, cocoa powder, and coconut are all keto-friendly. So if you're a chocoholic and can't keep away from the stuff, good news! You don't have to. Chocolate that's darker than 85% is actually allowed on keto in small amounts, and this is what goes into making keto-friendly desserts. So spoil yourself with decadent desserts like a Masala Chai Tea Latte (page 260) or a Strawberry and Mint Smoothie (page 263). These desserts won't kick you out of ketosis, so you can treat your sweet tooth guilt-free.

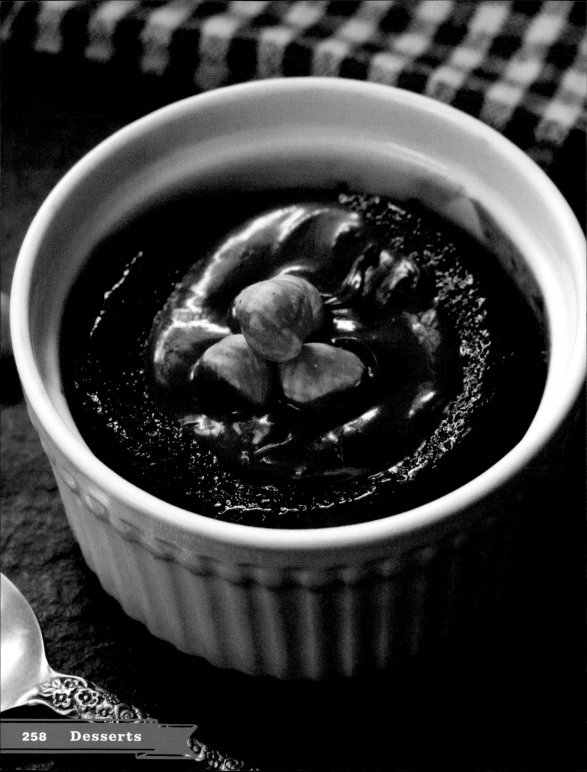

Hazelnut Microwave Mug Cake

YIELD: 2 SERVINGS • PREP TIME: 2 MINUTES • COOK TIME: 1 MINUTE
NUTRITIONAL INFO: CALORIES: 276 • FAT: 28G • NET CARBS: 2G • PROTEIN: 6G

This mug cake is quick, easy, and decadent thanks to the chocolate and hazelnut.

1 Mix all ingredients in a microwave-safe bowl or mug and microwave on high for 1 minute.

2 Let cool and serve.

INGREDIENTS

3 tablespoons hazelnut butter

1 tablespoon cocoa powder

1 tablespoon butter

1 tablespoon heavy whipping cream

1 egg

½ teaspoon baking powder

½ teaspoon vanilla extract

Stevia, to taste

Masala Chai Tea Latte

YIELD: 2 SERVINGS • PREP TIME: ABOUT 5 MINUTES
COOK TIME: 2 TO 3 MINUTES
NUTRITIONAL INFO: CALORIES: 52 • FAT: 6G • NET CARBS: 0G • PROTEIN: 0G

Indian milk tea spiced with ginger and cardamom makes for a satisfying dessert.

INGREDIENTS

2-inch piece ginger

4 cardamom pods

Pinch of fresh ground black pepper

cinnamon stick

1¾ cups water

2 tablespoons black tea

Sweetener of choice, to taste (optional)

2 tablespoons heavy whipping cream

1 Peel and chop the ginger and crush the cardamom. Place the ginger, cardamon, and pepper in a mortar and grind with a pestle.

2 In a small saucepan, combine water, ground spices, and cinnamon stick and bring to a boil.

3 Add the tea leaves and boil for 2 to 3 minutes. If desired, add in the sweetener of your choice.

4 Add cream to saucepan, stir well, then turn off the heat and let the tea sit for 1 to 2 minutes. Strain the tea into cups and serve.

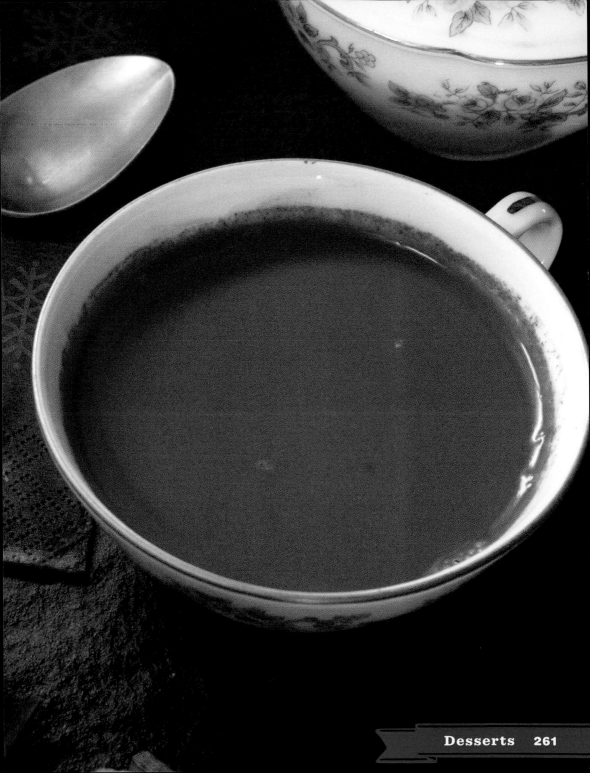

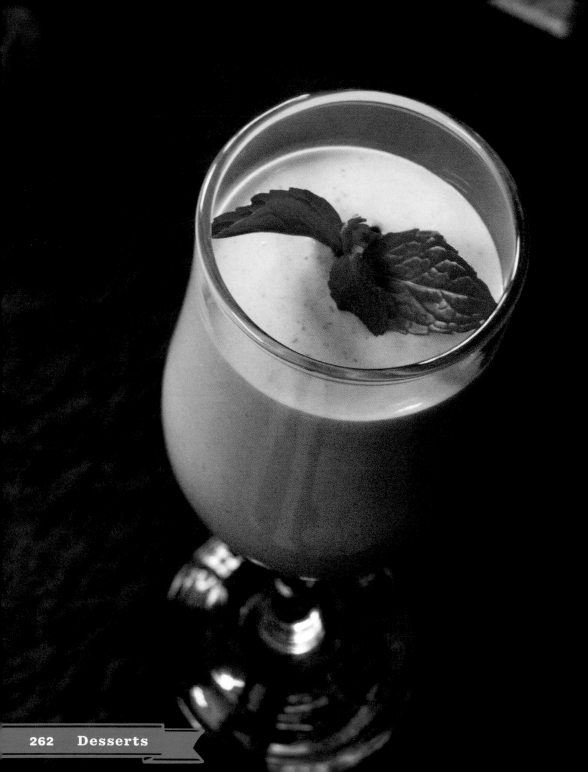

Strawberry and Mint Smoothie

YIELD: 2 SERVINGS • PREP TIME: 2 MINUTES
NUTRITIONAL INFO: CALORIES: 291 • FAT: 30G • NET CARBS: 5G • PROTEIN: 2G

A thick and refreshing keto smoothie.

1 Blend the strawberries with the cream cheese and mint leaves.

2 Add in the cream, coconut milk, and stevia and blend together.

3 Serve and garnish with mint.

INGREDIENTS

½ cup strawberries, sliced, stems removed

3½ teaspoons cream cheese

3 fresh mint leaves, plus more for garnish

3¼ oz. heavy whipping cream

½ cup unsweetened coconut milk

Stevia, to taste

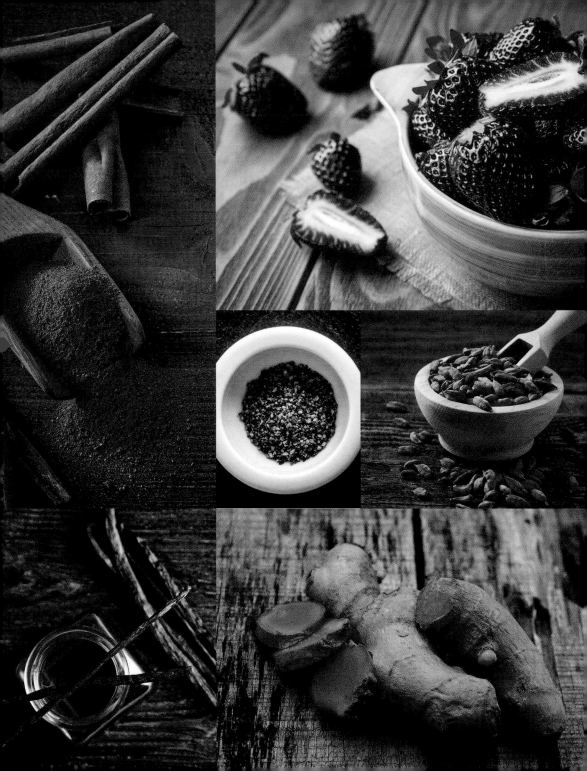

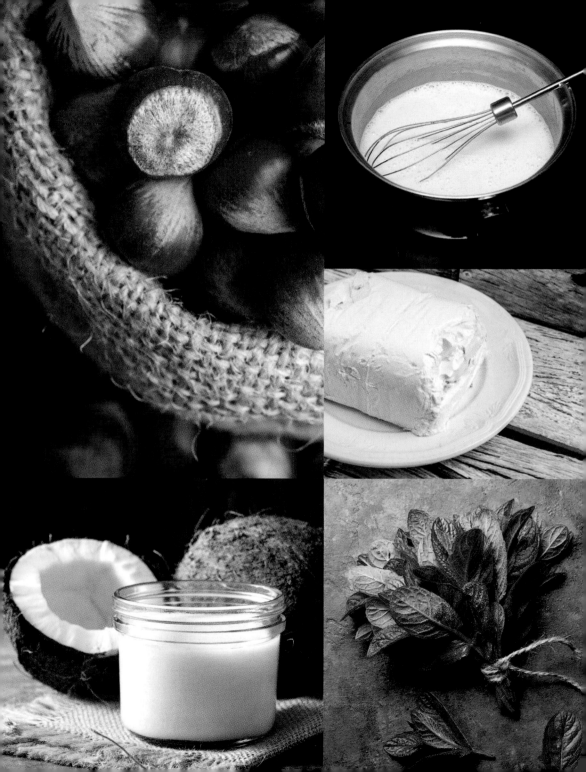

Index

Recipe and Image Credits

Recipes by Sahil Makhija:

Bacon and Cheese Omelet (24), Vietnamese Egg Coffee (35), Crustless Quiche (39), Coconut Flour Waffles (45), Butter Chicken Bites (54), Chicken Liver Pate (57), Lemon Pepper Chicken Wings (58), Peanut Butter Chicken Skewers (61), Crispy Fried Okra (71), Curried Kale Chips (72), Lemon Pepper Paneer (82), Chicken Noodles (85), Caprese Salad (95), Pesto & Feta Salad with Calamari and Chorizo (102), Basil Pesto (105), Roasted Bell Pepper Dip (109), Beef and Broccoli Stir Fry (147), Tenderloin Steak with Herbed Butter (163), Pork Chili Fry (170), Thai-Style Fried Rice (176), Creamy Pork Tenderloin (187), Chicken Fried Rice (192), Chili-Tomato Grilled Red Snapper (214), Pan-Seared Salmon in Bell Pepper Sauce (224), Yellow Thai Fish Curry (231), Indian-Chinese Hakka Noodles (240), Pesto Zoodles with Mushrooms and Olives (243), Vegetarian Thai Curry (244), Zucchini Carbonara (247), Hazelnut Microwave Cake (259), Masala Chai Tea Latte (260), Strawberry and Mint Smoothie (263)

Images courtesy of Sahil Makhija:

24, 34, 38, 44, 54-55, 56, 59, 60, 70-71, 73, 83, 84, 95, 108, 146, 162, 171, 177, 187, 193, 225, 230, 241, 242, 246, 258, 261, 262

All other images are used under official license from Shutterstock.com.

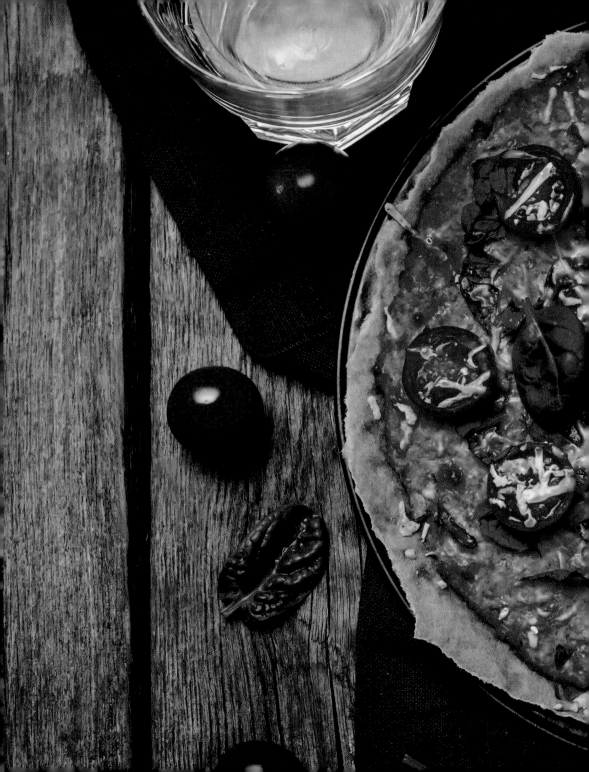

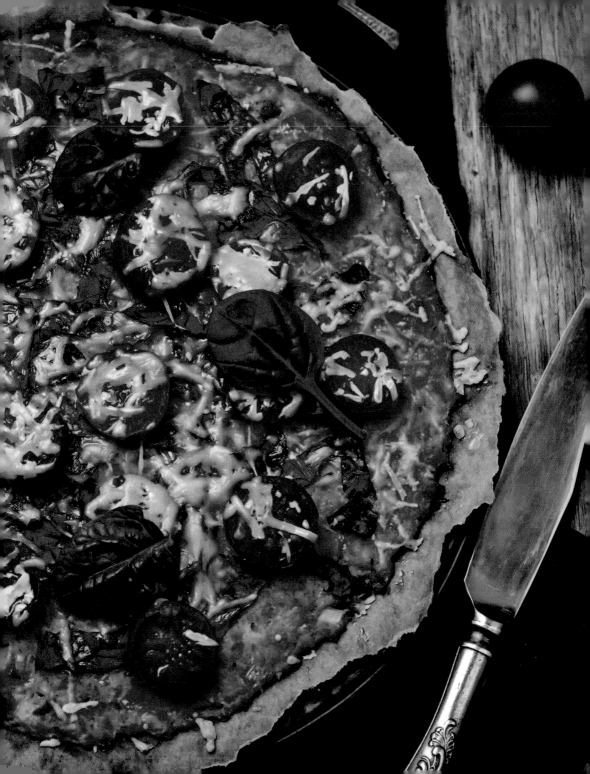

ABOUT CIDER MILL PRESS BOOK PUBLISHERS

Good ideas ripen with time. From seed to harvest, Cider Mill Press brings fine reading, information, and entertainment together between the covers of its creatively crafted books. Our Cider Mill bears fruit twice a year, publishing a new crop of titles each spring and fall.

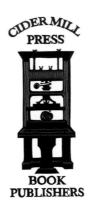

"Where Good Books Are Ready for Press"

VISIT US ONLINE:
www.cidermillpress.com

OR WRITE TO US AT
PO Box 454
12 Spring St.
Kennebunkport, Maine 04046